Pock
Prescriber

2012

Edited by

Timothy RJ Nicholson MBBS BSc MSc MRCP MRCPSYCH
Academic Clinical Lecturer, Section of Cognitive Neuropsychiatry,
Institute of Psychiatry, London, UK

Donald RJ Singer BMEDBIOL MD FRCP
Professor of Clinical Pharmacology and Therapeutics,
Clinical Sciences Research, Warwick Medical School,
University of Warwick and
University Hospitals Coventry and Warwickshire, Coventry, UK

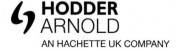
HODDER
ARNOLD
AN HACHETTE UK COMPANY

First published in Great Britain in 2004
Second edition 2006
Third edition 2009
Fourth edition published in 2011
This fifth edition published in 2012 by
Hodder Arnold, an imprint of Hodder Education, an Hachette UK Company,
338 Euston Road, London NW1 3BH

http://www.hoddereducation.com

British Library Cataloguing in Publication Data
A catalogue record for this book is available from the British Library

Library of Congress Cataloging-in-Publication Data
A catalog record for this book is available from the Library of Congress

ISBN-13 978 1 444 16316 2

1 2 3 4 5 6 7 8 9 10

Commissioning Editor: Caroline Makepeace
Project Editor: Stephen Clausard
Production Controller: Joanna Walker
Cover Designer: Peter Banks
Index: Merrall-Ross International Ltd

Typeset by Datapage India Pvt Ltd
Printed and bound in Spain

What do you think about this book? Or any other Hodder Arnold title?
Please visit our website: www.hodderarnold.com

CONTENTS

CONTRIBUTORS

Adam MC Archibald BSc(Hons) MBChB
StR Obstetrics and Gynaecology, NHS Greater Glasgow and Clyde

Peter J Barnes DM DSc FRCP FMedSci FRS
Professor and Consultant in Respiratory Medicine, National Heart & Lung Institute, Imperial College London

Alison Bedlow BSc MBBS FRCP DipRCPath
Consultant Dermatologist, South Warwickshire NHS Foundation Trust

Aodhan Breathnach MD FRCPath
Consultant Medical Microbiologist, Department of Medical Microbiology St George's Hospital, London

Emma C Derrett-Smith BSc MBBS MRCP
Clinical Research Fellow, Centre for Rheumatology and Connective Tissue Diseases, UCL Medical School, London

Timothy WR Doulton BSc MD MRCP
Consultant Nephrologist, Kent Kidney Care Centre, East Kent Hospitals University NHS Foundation Trust

David Hall BSc(Hons) MBChB(Hons)
Royal Air Force Medical Office

H Nikki Hall MBChB BSc(Hons)
Specialist Trainee in Ophthalmology, Queen Margaret Hospital, Dunfermline

Beth D Harrison MA BM BCh DM(Oxon) FRCP FRCPath
Consultant Haematologist, University Hospital Coventry and Warwickshire NHS Trust

Steven Harsum MBBS BSc PhD FRCOphth
Consultant Ophthalmologist, Epsom & St Helier University Hospitals NHS Trust

Robin DC Kumar BSc MBBS FRCA
Specialist Registrar in Anaesthesia and Intensive Care, King's College Hospital, London

Pete Maskell MBBS FRCP MSc
Consultant Stroke Physician and Elderly Care Lead, Maidstone and Tunbridge Wells NHS Trust

Allison C Morton BMedSci MBChB MRCP PhD
Consultant Cardiologist, Sheffield Teaching Hospitals NHS Foundation Trust; and Clinical Research Manager, NIHR Cardiovascular Biomedical Research Unit, Northern General Hospital, Sheffield

Victor Pace FRCP
Consultant in Palliative Medicine, St Christopher's Hospice, Sydenham, London

James JH Rucker MBBS BSc MRCPsych
Clinical Research Fellow, Social, Genetic and Developmental Psychiatry Centre, Institute of Psychiatry, King's College London and Honorary Specialist Registrar in General Adult Psychiatry, The South London and Maudsley NHS Foundation Trust, London

Stephen Derek Quinn MB BS BSc MRCOG
Clinical Research Fellow, St Mary's Hospital, London

Biba Stanton BMedSci MBBS MRCP PhD
Specialist Registrar, National Hospital for Neurology and Neurosurgery, Queen Square, London

Alex Tulloch PhD MRCP MRCPsych
BRC Preparatory Clinician Scientist Fellow

Esther Unitt BMedSci MBBS MRCP DM
Consultant Gastroenterologist and Hepatologist at the University Hospital, Coventry and Warwickshire Hospitals NHS Trust

W Stephen Waring BMedSci MB PhD FRCP(Edin)
Consultant in Acute Medicine, York Teaching Hospital NHS Foundation Trust, and Honorary Senior Lecturer, Hull York Medical School

FOREWORD

Contemporary medical practice necessitates a broad knowledge of drug treatments, which are constantly being updated and modified. I am delighted to write the foreword for this volume which, in the principle of the very best travel guides, is small but packed with essential and easily accessible information. Of all the subjects that are in the medical curriculum, pharmacology can sometimes seem especially abstract and theoretical. A quick flick through the pages of this book that are relevant to one's own speciality is an immediate reminder of the importance of understanding the ways in which the drugs that we routinely prescribe are handled. The clear identification of hazardous side effects and potential interactions is especially welcome. Finally, the section providing current information and management guidelines for commonly encountered medical emergencies is both clear and comprehensive.

Safe use of the modern therapeutic armamentarium is a daunting task for junior doctors and medical students. Although there has been a large growth in electronic resources and some excellent online textbooks have been produced, there remains a critical need for small reference texts that can be carried at all times and used to check drug doses or potential interactions at the point of prescription. The simple precaution of checking facts in any unfamiliar prescribing situation is likely to prevent mistakes, and exemplifies current emphasis on safe-practice and clinical risk management.

I believe that even the most senior specialist could learn something from this book's pages and that a comprehensive up-to-date volume such as this is an essential part of any junior doctor's tool kit, and will prove useful far beyond its target audience.

Professor Dame Carol M. Black DBE
Former president of the Royal College of Physicians

ACKNOWLEDGEMENTS

This book is dedicated to my family and friends as well as all the inspirational teachers I have been lucky enough to learn from over the years, in particular John Youle, Katie Blackman, Jerry Kirk, Carol Black, Huw Beynon, Martin Rossor, Michael Trimble, Maria Ron, Matthew Hotopf and Tony David.

Particular thanks for their help and time to Anand and Subbu, Usman Ali, Charlie Archer, Houman Ashrafian, Selma Aybek, Prithwish Bannerjee, Amlan Basu, Nick Bateman, Simone Brackenborough, Harris Birthright, Gurpreet Chana, Reena Chauhan, Roger Cross, Jonny Crowston, Chris Denton, Samantha Dickinson, Paul Dilworth, Michael Duick, Phil Dyer, Nick Eynon-Lewis, Fahad Farooqi, Catherine Farrow, Roger Fernandes, Arosha Fernando, Denise Forth, Jack Galliford, Thomas Galliford, Hamid Ghodse, Natasha Gilani, Caroline Goh, Nikesh Gudka, Ashan Gunarathne, Nadya Hamedi, Jane Henderson, Peter Hargreaves, Nicholas Hirsch, Rick Holliman, Emily Horwill, Saadhiya Hussain, Nick Jackson, Sudhesh Kumar, Simon Little, Ruey-Leng Loo, Graham MacGregor, Mel Mahadevan, Omar Malik, Janada Mamza, Chung Man Wan, Joela Matthews, Narbeh Melikian, Hina Mistry, Neil Muchatuta, Dev Mukerjee, Tejal Patel, Rahul Patel, Rakita Patel, Gideon Paul, Annabel Price, Deirdre Prinsloo, Gemma Robinson, Ricardo Sainz, Sailesh Sankar, Muriel Shannon, Amar Sharif, Jennifer Sharp, Ramsay Singer, Bran Sivakumar, Sian Stanley, Richard Stratton, Henry Squire, Becky Szekely, Sheena Thomas, Mike Travis, Rudolf Uher, Aaron Vallance, Payal Vasani, Jim Wade, Mandy Wan, Jayne Yeung and Abbas Zaidi.

Special thanks to Helen Galley.

The information in this book has been collated from many sources, including manufacturer's information sheets ('SPCs' – Summary of Product Characteristics sheets), the *British National Formulary* (BNF), national and international guidelines, as well as numerous pharmacology and general medical books, journals and papers. Where information is not consistent between these sources, that from the SPCs has generally been taken as definitive.

HOW TO USE THIS BOOK

STANDARD LAYOUT OF DRUGS
DRUG/TRADE NAME

Class/action: More information is given for generic forms, especially for the original and most commonly used drug(s) of each class.

Use: use^x (correlating to dose as below).

CI: contraindications; **L** (liver failure), **R** (renal failure), **H** (heart failure), **P** (pregnancy), **B** (breastfeeding). *Allergy to active drug, or any excipients (other substances in the preparation) assumed too obvious to mention.*

Caution: **L** (liver failure), **R** (renal failure), **H** (heart failure), **P** (pregnancy), **B** (breastfeeding), **E** (elderly patients). If a contraindication is given for a drug it is assumed too obvious to mention that a caution is also inherently implied.

SE: side effects; listed in order of frequency encountered. Common/important side effects set in **bold**.

Warn: information to give to patients before starting drug.

Monitor: parameters that need to be monitored during treatment.

Interactions: included only if very common or potentially serious; ↑/↓**P450** (induces/inhibits cytochrome P450 metabolism), **W+** (increases effect of warfarin), **W−** (decreases effect of warfarin).

Dose: dose^x (for Use^x as above). *NB Doses are for adults only.*

Important points highlighted at end of drug entry.

Use/dose^{NICE}: National Institute of Health and Clinical Excellence guidelines exist for the drug (basics often in BNF – see www.nice.org.uk for full details).

Dose$^{BNF/SPC}$: dose regimen complicated; please refer to BNF and/or SPC (Summary of Product Characteristics sheet; the manufacturer's information sheet enclosed with drug packaging – can also be viewed at or downloaded from www.emc.medicines.org.uk).

Asterisks (*) and **daggers (†)** denote links between information within local text.

> **Only relevant sections are included** for each drug. **Trade names** (in OUTLINE font) are given only if found regularly on drug charts or if non-proprietary (generic, non-trade-name) drug does not exist yet.

KEY

 Potential dangers highlighted with skull and cross-bones

▼ New drug or new indication under intense surveillance by Committee on Safety of Medicines (CSM): *important to report all suspected drug reactions via Yellow Card scheme* (accurate as going to press: from December 2011 CSM list)

☺ *Good for*: reasons to give a certain drug when choice exists

☹ *Bad for*: reasons to not give a certain drug when choice exists

⇒ Causes/goes to

∴ Therefore

Δ Change/disturbance

Ψ Psychiatric

↑ Increase/high

↓ Decrease/low

> ↑/↓ electrolytes refers to serum levels, unless stated otherwise.

DOSES

od	once daily	nocte	at night
bd	twice daily	mane	in the morning
tds	three times daily	prn	as required
qds	four times daily	stat	at once

ROUTES

im	intramuscular	po	oral
inh	inhaled	pr	rectal
iv	intravenous	sc	subcutaneous
ivi	intravenous infusion	top	topical
neb	via nebuliser	sl	sublingual

> Routes are presumed po, unless stated otherwise.

LIST OF ABBREVIATIONS

5-ASA	5-aminosalicylic acid
5HT	5-hydroxytryptamine (= serotonin)
A&E	accident and emergency
AAC	antibiotic-associated colitis
Ab	antibody
ABPM	ambulatory blood pressure monitoring
ACC	American College of Cardiology
ACCP	American College of Chest Physicians
ACE-i	ACE inhibitor
ACh	acetylcholine
ACS	acute coronary syndrome
ADP	adenosine phosphate
AF	atrial fibrillation
Ag	antigen
AHA	American Heart Association
AKI	acute kidney injury
ALL	acute lymphoblastic leukaemia
ALP	alkaline phosphatase
ALS	adult life support (algorithms of European Resuscitation Council)
ALT	alanine(-amino) transferase
AMI	acute myocardial infarction
AMTS	abbreviated mental test score (same as MTS)
ANA	anti-nuclear antigens
APTT	activate partial thromboplastin time
ARB(s)	angiotensin receptor blocker(s)
ARDS	adult respiratory distress syndrome
AS	aortic stenosis
ASAP	as soon as possible
assoc	associated
AST	aspartate transaminase
AV	arteriovenous

AVM	arteriovenous malformation
AVN	atrioventricular node
AZT	zidovudine
BBB	bundle branch block
BCSH	British Committee for Standards in Haematology
BCT	broad complex tachycardia
BF	blood flow
BG	serum blood glucose in mmol/l; *see also CBG*
BHS	British Hypertension Society
BIH	benign intracranial hypertension
BIPAP	bilevel/biphasic positive airway pressure
BM	bone marrow (NB: BM is often used, confusingly, to signify finger-prick glucose; CBG (capillary blood glucose) is used for this purpose in this book)
BMI	body mass index = weight (kg)/height $(m)^2$
BP	blood pressure
BPH	benign prostatic hypertrophy
BTS	British Thoracic Society
Bx	biopsy
C	constipation
Ca	cancer (NB: calcium is abbreviated to Ca^{2+})
CAH	congenital adrenal hyperplasia
CBF	cerebral blood flow
CBG	capillary blood glucose in mmol/l (finger-prick testing) (NB: BM is often used to denote this, but this is confusing and less accurate and thus not used in this book)
CCF	congestive cardiac failure
cf	compared with
CI	contraindicated
CK	creatine kinase
CKD	chronic kidney disease
CLL	chronic lymphocytic leukaemia
CML	chronic myelogenous leukaemia
CMV	cytomegalovirus

CNS	central nervous system
CO	cardiac output
COPD	chronic obstructive pulmonary disease
COX	cyclo-oxygenase
CPR	cardiopulmonary resuscitation
CRF	chronic renal failure
CRP	C reactive protein
CSF	cerebrospinal fluid
CSM	Committee on Safety of Medicines
CT	computerised tomography
CVA	cerebrovascular accident
CVP	central venous pressure
CXR	chest X-ray
D	diarrhoea
D&V	diarrhoea and vomiting
$D_{1/2/3 \dots}$	dopamine receptor subtype 1/2/3 ...
DA	dopamine
DCT	distal convoluted tubule
dfx	defects
DI	diabetes insipidus
DIC	disseminated intravascular coagulation
DIGAMI	glucose, insulin and potassium intravenous infusion used in acute myocardial infarction
DKA	diabetic ketoacidosis
DM	diabetes mellitus
DMARD	disease-modifying anti-rheumatoid arthritis drug
dt	due to
DWI	diffusion weighted (imaging); specialist MRI mostly used for stroke/TIA
Dx	diagnosis
EØ	eosinophils
e'lyte	electrolyte
EBV	Epstein–Barr virus
ECG	electrocardiogram
ECT	electroconvulsive therapy

EF	ejection fraction
ENT	ear, nose and throat
EPSE	extrapyramidal side effects
ERC	European Resuscitation Council
ESC	European Society of Cardiology
ESR	erythrocyte sedimentation rate
exac	exacerbates
FBC	full blood count
Fe	iron
FFP	fresh frozen plasma
FHx	family history
FiO_2	inspired O_2 concentration
FMF	familial Mediterranean fever
fx	effects
G6PD	glucose-6-phosphate dehydrogenase
GABA	gamma aminobutyric acid
GBS	Guillain–Barré syndrome
GCS	Glasgow Coma Scale
GFR	glomerular filtration rate
GI	gastrointestinal
GIK	glucose, insulin and K^+ infusion
GMC	General Medical Council (of UK)
GTN	glyceryl trinitrate
GU	genitourinary
h	hour(s)
H(O)CM	hypertrophic (obstructive) cardiomyopathy
Hb	haemoglobin
HB	heart block
HBPM	home blood pressure monitoring
Hct	haematocrit
HDL	high density lipoprotein
HF	heart failure
HIV	human immunodeficiency virus
HLA	human leucocyte antigen
HMG-CoA	3-hydroxy-3-methyl-glutaryl coenzyme A

HONK	hyperosmolar non-ketotic state
hrly	hourly
HSV	herpes simplex virus
HTN	hypertension
HUS	haemolytic uraemic syndrome
Hx	history
IBD	inflammatory bowel disease
IBS	irritable bowel syndrome
ICP	intracranial pressure
ICU	intensive care unit
IHD	ischaemic heart disease
IL-2	interleukin 2
im	intramuscular
inc	including
inh	inhaled
INR	international normalised ratio (prothrombin ratio)
IOP	intraocular pressure
ITP	immune/idiopathic thrombocytopenic purpura
ITU	intensive therapy unit
iv	intravenous
IVDU	intravenous drug user
ivi	intravenous infusion
Ix	investigation
K^+	potassium (serum levels unless stated otherwise)
LØ	lymphocytes
LA	long-acting
LBBB	left bundle branch block
LDL	low density lipoprotein
LF	liver failure
LFTs	liver function tests
LMWH	low-molecular-weight heparin
LP	lumbar puncture
LVF	left ventricular failure
MØ	macrophages
mane	in morning

MAOI	monoamine oxidase inhibitor
MAP	mean arterial pressure
MCA	middle cerebral artery
MCV	mean corpuscular volume
metab	metabolised
MG	myasthenia gravis
MHRA	Medicines and Healthcare Products Regulatory Authority (UK)
MI	myocardial infarction
MMF	mycophenolate mofetil
MMSE	Mini-Mental State Examination (scored out of 30[*])
MR	modified-release (drug preparation)[†]
MRI	magnetic resonance imaging
MRSA	methicillin-resistant *Staphylococcus aureus*
MS	multiple sclerosis
MTS	(abbreviated) Mental Test Score (scored out of 10*)
MUST	malnutrition universal screening tool
Mx	management
N	nausea
N&V	nausea and vomiting
NØ	neutrophils
NA	noradrenaline (norepinephrine)
Na[1]	sodium (serum levels unless stated otherwise)
NBM	nil by mouth
NCT	narrow complex tachycardia
NDRI	noradrenaline and dopamine reuptake inhibitor
neb	via nebuliser
NGT	nasogastric tube
NH	non-Hodgkin's (lymphoma)
NIHSS	National (US) Institute of Health Stroke Scale
NIV	non-invasive ventilation
NMJ	neuromuscular junction
NMS	neuroleptic malignant syndrome
NPIS	National Poisons Information Service
NSAID	nonsteroidal anti-inflammatory drug

NSTEMI	non-ST elevation myocardial infarction
NYHA	New York Heart Association
OCD	obsessive compulsive disorder
OCP	oral contraceptive pill
OD	overdose *(NB: od = once daily!)*
OGD	oesophagogastroduodenoscopy
p'way(s)	pathway(s)
PAN	polyarteritis nodosa
PBC	primary biliary cirrhosis
PCI	percutaneous coronary intervention (now preferred term for percutaneous transluminal coronary angioplasty (PTCA), which is a subtype of PCI)
PCOS	polycystic ovary syndrome
PCP	*Pneumocystis carinii* pneumonia
PCV	packed cell volume
PDA	patent ductus arteriosus
PE	pulmonary embolism
PEA	pulseless electrical activity
PEG	percutaneous endoscopic gastrostomy
PG(x)	prostaglandin (receptor subtype x)
phaeo	phaeochromocytoma
PHx	past history (of)
PID	pelvic inflammatory disease
PML	progressive multifocal leukoencephalopathy
PMR	polymyalgia rheumatica
po	by mouth
PO$_4$	phosphate (serum levels, unless stated otherwise)
PPI	proton pump inhibitor
pr	rectal
prep(s)	preparation(s)
prn	as required
PSA	prostate specific antigen
Pt	platelet(s)
PT	prothrombin time
PTH	parathyroid hormone

PTSD	post-traumatic stress disorder
PU	peptic ulcer
PUO	pyrexia of unknown origin
PVD	peripheral vascular disease
Px	prophylaxis
QT(c)	QT interval (corrected for rate)
RA	rheumatoid arthritis
RAS	renal artery stenosis
RBF	renal blood flow
RF	renal failure
RLS	restless legs syndrome
ROSIER	recognition of stroke in emergency room scale for diagnosis of stroke/TIA
RR	respiratory rate
RRT	renal replacement therapy
RSV	respiratory syncytial virus
RTI	respiratory tract infection
RV	right ventricle
RVF	right ventricular failure
Rx	treatment
SAH	subarachnoid haemorrhage
SAN	sinoatrial node
SBE	subacute bacterial endocarditis
sc	subcutaneous
SE(s)	side effect(s)
sec	second(s)
SIGN	Scottish Intercollegiate Guidelines Network
SIADH	syndrome of inappropriate antidiuretic hormone
SJS	Stevens–Johnson syndrome
sl	sublingual
SLE	systemic lupus erythematosus
SOA	swelling of ankles
SOB (OE)	shortness of breath (on exertion)
SPC	summary of product characteristic sheet (see page viii)
spp	species

SR	slow/sustained release (drug preparation)
SSRI	selective serotonin reuptake inhibitor
SSS	sick sinus syndrome
STEMI	ST elevation myocardial infarction
supp	suppository
SVT	supraventricular tachycardia
$t_{1/2}$	half-life
T_3	triiodothyronine/liothyronine
T_4	thyroxine ($\uparrow$/ $\downarrow T_4$ = hyper/hypothyroid)
TCA	tricyclic antidepressant
TE	thromboembolism
TEDS	thromboembolism deterrent stockings
TEN	toxic epidermal necrolysis
TFTs	thyroid function tests
TG	triglyceride
TIBC	total iron binding capacity
TIMI score	risk score for UA/NSTEMI named after TIMI (thrombolysis in MI) trial
TNF	tumour necrosis factor
top	topical
TPMT	thiopurine methyltransferase
TPR	total peripheral resistance
TTA(s)	(drugs) to take away, i.e. prescriptions for inpatients on discharge/leave (aka TTO)
TTO(s)	see TTA
TTP	thrombotic thrombocytopenic purpura
U&Es	urea and electrolytes
UA(P)	unstable angina (pectoris)
UC	ulcerative colitis
URTI	upper respiratory tract infection
UTI	urinary tract infection
UV	ultraviolet
V	vomiting
VE(s)	ventricular ectopic(s)
VF	ventricular fibrillation

vit	vitamin
VLDL	very low density lipoprotein
VT	ventricular tachycardia
VTE	venous thromboembolism
VZV	varicella zoster virus (chickenpox/shingles)
w	with
w/in	within
w/o	without
WCC	white cell count
WE	Wernicke's encephalopathy
wk	week
WPW	Wolff–Parkinson–White syndrome
Wt	weight
xs	excess
ZE	Zollinger–Ellison syndrome

HOW TO PRESCRIBE SAFELY

Take time/care to ↓risk to patients (and protect yourself).
Always check the following are correct for all prescriptions: patient,
indication and drug, **legible** format (generic name, clarity, handwriting,
identifiable signature, your contact number), dosage, frequency, time(s)
of day, date, duration of treatment, route of administration.

DO

- Make a clear, accurate record in the notes of all medicines
  prescribed, written at the time of prescription
- Complete allergy box and alert labels, where relevant
- Include on all drug charts and TTAs the patient's surname and
  given name, date of birth, date of admission and consultant (if
  possible use a printed label for patient details)
- **PRINT** (i.e. use upper case) all drugs as approved (generic) names,
  e.g. 'IBUPROFEN' *not* 'nurofen'
- State dose, route and frequency, giving strength of solutions/creams
- Write the word microgram in full; avoid abbreviations such as mcg
  or μ
- Abbreviate the word gram to 'g' (rather than 'gm' which is easily
  confused with mg)
- Write the word 'units' in full, preceded by a space; abbreviating to
  'U' can be misread as zero (a 10-fold error)
- Document weight where dosing is weight-dependent
- Write quantities <1 g in mg (e.g. 400 mg *not* 0.4 g)
- Write quantities <1 mg in micrograms (e.g. 200 micrograms *not*
  0.2 mg).
- Not use trailing zeroes (10 mg *not* 10.0 mg)
- Precede decimal points with another figure (e.g 0.8 ml *not* .8 ml)
  and only use decimals where unavoidable
- Check and recheck calculations
- Provide clear additional instructions, e.g. for monitoring, review of
  antibiotic route and duration, maximum daily/24 h dose for PRN
  drugs

- Specify solution to be used and duration of any iv infusions/injections
- Avoid using abbreviated/non-standard drug names
- Avoid writing 'T' (tablet sign) for non-tablet formulations, e.g. sprays
- Amend a prescribed drug by drawing a line through it, date and initial this, then rewrite as new prescription
- Check and count number of drugs when rewriting a drug chart
- Check when prescribing unfamiliar drug(s)/doses or drugs you were familiar with but haven't prescribed recently.

IMPORTANT FURTHER ADVICE

1 Make sure choice of drug and dose is right for the patient, their condition and significant comorbidity, with particular attention to age*, gender, ethnicity, renal or liver dysfunction, risk of drug–drug and drug–disease interactions, and risks in pregnancy (and those of child-bearing age who may become pregnant) and during breastfeeding. Anticipate possible effects of over-the-counter and herbal medicines and lifestyle (e.g. dietary salt and alcohol intake).

*Although arbitrary age of >65 denotes 'elderly', fx of age can occur earlier/later and are continuous.

2 Common settings where drug problems occur are often predictable if you understand relevant pathology, routes of drug metabolism (liver, P450, renal, etc) and drug mechanisms of action. Take particular care with:

- Renal or liver disease
- Pregnancy/breastfeeding: use safest options (in the UK consider consulting the National Teratology Information Service; tel: 0191 232 1525)
- NSAIDs/bisphosphonates and peptic ulcer disease
- Asthma and β-blockers
- Conditions worsened by antimuscarinic drugs (see p. 233): urinary retention/BPH, glaucoma, paralytic ileus

- Rare conditions where drugs commonly pose risk, e.g. porphyria, myasthenia, G6PD deficiency, phaeo.

3 Always ensure informed consent; agree proposed prescriptions with the patient (or carer if patient has authorised their involvement in their care or has lost capacity), explaining proposed benefits, nature and duration of treatment, clarifying concerns, warning of possible, especially severe, adverse effects, highlighting recommended monitoring and review arrangements and stating what the patient should do in the event of a suspected adverse reaction. Only in extreme emergencies can it be justified to have not done this. For drugs with common potentially fatal/severe side effects document that these risks have been explained to, and accepted by, the patient.

4 See legal advice on eligibility to prescribe and use of unlicensed medicines on the GMC website (www.gmc-uk.org).

5 Make sure that you are being objective. Prescribing should be for the benefit of the patient not the prescriber.

6 Keep up to date about medicines you are prescribing and the related conditions you are treating.

7 Follow CSM guidance on reporting suspected adverse reactions to medicines (see top right link at www.mhra.gov.uk for links to details of the Yellow Card reporting scheme and downloads of reported adverse drug reactions for specific medicines).

8 Ensure continuity of care by keeping the patient's GP (or other preferred medical adviser) informed about prescribing, monitoring and follow-up arrangements and responsibilities.

9 Check that appropriate previous medicines are continued and over-the-counter and herbal medicine use is recorded.

10 Patient Group Directions: the GMC advises these should be limited to situations where there is a 'distinct advantage for patient care ... consistent with appropriate professional relationships and accountability'.

Common/useful drugs

ABCIXIMAB/REOPRO

Antiplatelet agent – monoclonal Ab against platelet glycoprotein IIb/IIIa receptor (involved in Pt aggregation).

Use: Px of ischaemic complications of PCI and Px of MI in unstable angina unresponsive to conventional Rx awaiting PCI[NICE] (see p. 240).

CI: active internal bleeding, CVA w/in 2 years, intracranial neoplasm, aneurysm or AVM. Major surgery, intracranial/intraspinal surgery or trauma w/in 2 months. Hypertensive retinopathy, vasculitis, ↓Pt, haemorrhagic diathesis, severe ↑BP. **L** (if severe)/**R** (if requiring haemodialysis)/**B**.

Caution: drugs that ↑bleeding risk, **L/R/P/E**.

SE: bleeding* /↓Pt*, N&V, ↓BP, ↓HR, pain (chest, back or pleuritic), headache, fever. Rarely, hypersensitivity, tamponade, ARDS.

Monitor: FBC* (baseline plus 2–4 h, 12 h and 24 h after giving) and clotting (baseline at least).

Dose: 250 microgram/kg iv over 1 min, then 0.125 microgram/kg/min (max 10 microgram/min) ivi; see BNF/product literature for dose timing. *NB: use iv non-pyrogenic, low protein binding filter. Needs concurrent heparin.* Specialist use only: get senior advice or contact on-call cardiology.

ACAMPROSATE/CAMPRAL EC

Modifies GABA transmission ⇒ ↓pleasurable fx of alcohol ∴ ↓s craving and relapse rate.

Use: maintaining alcohol abstinence.

CI: **L** (only if severe), **R/P/B**.

SE: GI upset, pruritus, rash, Δ libido.

Dose: 666 mg tds po if age 18–65 years (avoid outside this age range) and >60 kg (if <60 kg give 666 mg mane then 333 mg noon and nocte). *Start ASAP after alcohol stopped. Usually give for 1 year.*

ACARBOSE

Oral hypoglycaemic: α-glucosidase inhibitor. Delays digestion and ↓s absorption of starch and sucrose.

Use: DM not controlled by conventional oral hypoglycaemics.

CI: IBD, hernia, Hx of abdominal surgery or obstruction **R** (if severe) **L/P/B**.

SE: flatulence, GI upset, rarely hepatitis and ileus.

Monitor: LFTs.

Interactions: may ↑hypoglycaemic fx of sulphonylureas and insulin.

Dose: initially 50 mg od po, ↑up to 200 mg tds po.

ACIDEX

Alginate raft-forming oral suspension for acid reflux.

Dose: 10–20 ml after meals and at bedtime (NB: 3 mmol Na^+/5 ml)

ACETAZOLAMIDE/DIAMOX

Carbonic anhydrase inhibitor (sulphonamide).

Use: glaucoma (acute-angle closure, primary open-angle unresponsive to maximal topical Rx, or secondary), ↑ICP. Rarely for epilepsy or diuresis.

CI: ↓K^+, ↓Na^+, ↑Cl^- acidosis, sulphonamide allergy, adrenocortical insufficiency. **L** (if severe)/**R**.

Caution: acidosis, pulmonary obstruction **R/P/E**.

SE: nausea/GI upset, paraesthesia, drowsiness, mood Δ, headache, Δ LFTs. If prolonged use acidosis (metabolic) and e'lyte Δs. Rarely blood disorders and skin reactions (inc SJS/TENS).

Monitor: FBC, U&E if prolonged use.

Interactions: ↑s levels of carbamazepine. Can ↑cardiac toxicity (via ↓K^+) of disopyramide, flecainide, lidocaine and cardiac glycosides. ↓s fx of methenamine and ↑ fx of quinidine.

Dose: 0.25–1 g/day po or iv^{SPC}. Also available as 250 mg MR preparation (as Diamox SR; max 2 capsules/day).

☠ Extravasation at injection site can ⇒ necrosis ☠.

ACETYLCYSTEINE/PARVOLEX

Precursor of glutathione, which detoxifies metabolites of paracetamol.

Use: paracetamol OD.

Caution: asthma*.

SE: allergy: rash, bronchospasm*, anaphylactoid reactions (esp if ivi too quick**).
Dose: initially 150 mg/kg in 200 ml 5% glucose as ivi over 15 min, then 50 mg/kg in 500 ml over 4 h, then 100 mg/kg in 1 litre over 16 h. NB: use max weight of 110 kg for dose calculation, even if patient weighs more. Ensure not given too quickly**. See p. 266 for Mx of paracetamol OD and treatment line graph.

ACICLOVIR (previously ACYCLOVIR)

Antiviral. Inhibits DNA polymerase *only in infected cells*: needs activation by viral thymidine kinase (produced by herpes spp).
Use: *iv:* severe HSV or VZV infections, e.g. meningitis, encephalitis and in immunocompromised patients (esp HIV – also used for Px); *po/top:* mucous membrane, genital, eye infections.
Caution: dehydration*, **R/P/B**.
SE: at ↑doses: **AKI, encephalopathy** (esp if dehydrated*). Also **hypersensitivity**, seizures, GI upset, blood disorders, skin reactions (including photosensitivity), headache, many non-specific neurological symptoms, ↓Pt, ↓WBC. Rarely Ψ reactions and hepatotoxicity.
Interactions: levels ↑d by probenecid.
Dose: 5 mg/kg tds ivi over 1 h (10 mg/kg if HSV encephalitis or VZV in immunocompromised patients); po/top^SPC/BNF.

☠ ivi leaks ⇒ severe local inflammation/ulceration ☠.

ACTIVATED CHARCOAL see Charcoal.

ACTRAPID Short-acting soluble insulin; see p. 202 for use.

ADENOSINE

Purine nucleoside. Slows AVN conduction time, dilates coronary arteries; acts on its own specific receptors.
Use: Rx of paroxysmal SVT (esp if accessory p'ways e.g. WPW) and Dx of SVT (NCT or BCT; ↓s rate to reveal underlying rhythm).
CI: ☠ asthma* (consider verapamil instead).☠ 2nd-/3rd-degree AV block or sick sinus syndrome (if either w/o pacemaker).

Caution: heart transplant (↓dose), AF/atrial flutter (↑s accessory pathway conduction), ↑QTc, COPD*.

SE: bronchospasm*, ↓BP. Rarely ↓HR/asystole/arrhythmias (mostly transient), angina (discontinue if occurs) & flushing.

Warn: can ⇒ transient unpleasant feelings: facial flushing, dyspnoea, choking feeling, nausea, chest pain and light-headedness.

Interactions: fx ↑by **dipyridamole**: ↓initial adenosine dose to 0.5–1 mg and watch for ↑bleeding (*anti-Pt fx of dipyridamole also ↑d by adenosine*). fx ↓d by **theophyllines** and caffeine. Use with digoxin may ↑risk of VF.

Dose: 3–6 mg iv over 2 sec; double dose and repeat every 1–2 min until response or significant AV block (max 12 mg/dose). *NB: attach cardiac monitor and give via central (or large peripheral) vein, then flush.* $t_{1/2}$ <10 sec: often needs readministration (esp if given for Rx cf Dx).

ADRENALINE (im/iv)

Sympathomimetic: powerful stimulation of α (vasoconstriction), β_1(↑HR, ↑contractility) and β_2 (vasodilation, bronchodilation, uterine relaxation). Also ↓s immediate mast cell cytokine release.

Use: CPR and anaphylaxis (see algorithms on inside and outside front cover, respectively). Rarely for other causes of bronchospasm or shock (e.g. 2° to spinal/epidural anaesthesia).

Caution: cerebrovascular* and heart disease (esp arrhythmias and HTN), DM, ↑T_4, glaucoma (angle closure), labour (esp 2nd stage), phaeo. **H/E**.

SE: ↑HR, ↑BP, anxiety, sweats, tremor, headache, peripheral vasoconstriction, arrhythmias, pulmonary oedema (at ↑doses), N&V, weakness, dizziness, Ψ disturbance, hyperglycaemia, urinary retention (esp if ↑prostate), local reactions. Rarely CVA* (2° to HTN: monitor BP).

Interactions: fx ↑d by dopexamine, TCAs, ergotamine and oxytocin. Risk of: 1. ↑↑BP and ↓HR with non-cardioselective β-blockers (can also ⇒ ↓HR), TCAs, MAOIs and moclobemide. 2. arrhythmias with digoxin, quinidine and volatile liquid anaesthetics (e.g. halothane) and TCAs. Avoid use with tolazine or rasagiline.

Dose: CPR: 1 mg iv = 10 ml of 1 in **10 000** (100 microgram/ml) then flush with ≥20 ml saline. If no or delayed iv access, try intraosseous route and, if this is not possible, give 2–3 mg via endotracheal tube diluted to 10 ml with sterile water. Repeat as per ALS algorithm (see front cover). **Anaphylaxis:** 0.5 mg im (or sc) = 0.5 ml of 1 in **1000** (1 mg/ml); repeat after 5 min if no response. (If cardiac arrest seems imminent or concerns over im absorption, give 0.5 mg iv slowly = 5 ml of 1 in **10 000** (100 microgram/ml) at 1 ml/min until response – get senior help first if possible as iv route ⇒ ↑risk of arrhythmias.)

☠ Don't confuse 1 in 1000 (im) with 1:10 000 (iv) solutions ☠.

ADVIL see Ibuprofen.

AGGRASTAT see Tirofiban; IIb/IIIa inhibitor (anti-Pt drug) for IHD.

▼ AGOMELATINE/VALDOXAN

Antidepressant: synthetic melatonin analogue; melatonin receptor (MT1/MT2) agonist (also $5HT_{2C/B}$ antagonist); no effect on monoamine reuptake; resynchronises circadian rhythms and ↑s NA/DA in frontal cortex via $5HT_{2C}$ antagonism.

Use: depression; esp if risk of inconsistent use (low risk of withdrawal syndrome on discontinuation) or if prominent insomnia/sleep reversal.

CI: dementia **L/B**.

Caution: elderly, history of mania (bipolar). **R/P/E**.

SE: nausea, diarrhoea, constipation, abdo pain, ΔLFTs (↑ transaminases in 5%; usually transient), drowsiness, headache, sweating, anxiety, suicidal behaviour.

Monitor: LFTs before and 6, 12 and 24 wks after starting.

Interactions: levels ↑↑ by strong CYP1A2 inhibitors (e.g. fluvoxamine, ciprofloxacin – avoid) and ↑ by moderate inhibitors (e.g. propranolol, enoxacin). ↑ risk of convulsions with atomoxetine. Avoid with artemether/lumefantrine.

Dose: 25 mg nocte (can ↑ to 50 mg nocte after 2 wks).

ALENDRONATE (ALENDRONIC ACID)/FOSAMAX

Bisphosphonate: ↓s osteoclastic bone resorption.

Use: osteoporosis Rx and Px (esp if on corticosteroids).

CI: delayed GI emptying (esp achalasia and oesophageal stricture/other abnormalities), ↓Ca^{2+}, unable to sit/stand upright ≥30 min, **R**(if severe)/**P**/**B**.

Caution: upper GI disorders (inc gastritis/PU) **R**.

SE: oesophageal reactions*, GI upset/distension, ↓Ca^{2+}, ↓PO_4^{2-} (transient), PU, hypersensitivity (esp skin reactions), myalgia. Rarely osteonecrosis and femoral stress fractures (discontinue drug and should receive no further bisphosphonates).

Warn: take with full glass of water on an empty stomach ≥30 min before, and stay upright until breakfast*. Stop tablets and seek medical attention if symptoms of oesophageal irritation develop.

Dose: 10 mg mane[SPC/BNF] (10 mg od dosing can be given as once-wkly 70-mg tablet *if for post-menopausal osteoporosis*).

ALFACALCIDOL

1-α-hydroxycholecalciferol: partially activated vitamin D (1α hydroxy group normally added by kidney), but still requires hepatic (25)-hydroxylation for full activation.

Use: severe vitamin D deficiency 2° to CRF.

CI/SE: ↑Ca^{2+}

Caution: nephrolithiasis, **E**.

Monitor: Ca^{2+}: monitor levels wkly, watch for symptoms (esp N&V), rash, nephrocalcinosis.

Interactions: fx may be ↓d by barbiturates and anticonvulsants.

Dose: initially 1 microgram (=1000 nanograms) od po; maintenance 250–1000 nanograms od po.

NB: ↓dose in elderly (initial dose 500 nanograms).

▼ ALISKIREN

Direct renin inhibitor (↓s angiotensinogen ⇒ angiotensin I).

Use: essential HTN (*for advice on stepped HTN Mx see p. 182*).

CI: potent P-glycoprotein inhibitors (*ciclosporin, verapamil, quinidine) **P**/**B**.

Caution: dehydration (risk of ↓BP), RAS, diuretics, ↓Na^+ diet, ** ↑K^+, moderate potent P-glycoprotein inhibitors (*keto-/itra-conazole, clari-/teli-/ery-thromycin, amiodarone), DM***, **R**(if GFR <30 ml/min) /**H**/**P**/**B**/**E**.

SE: diarrhoea, dizziness, ↓BP, ↑K^+, ↓GFR. Rarely rash, angioedema, ↓Hb.

Monitor: U&Es esp ** ↑K^+ if taking ACE-i, ARBs, K^+ sparing diuretics, K^+ salts (inc dietary salt substitutes) or heparin. Check BG/HbA_{1C} regularly***.

Interactions: metab by/ ↓/↑P450 ∴ many; ↓s furosemide levels. Levels ↓ by irbesartan; levels ↑ by keto-/itra-conazole. fx ↓ by ↓Na^+ diet and NSAIDs. fx ↑ by P-glycoprotein inhibitors (see *CI/Caution).

Dose: initially 150 mg od, ↑ing to 300 mg od if required.

ALLOPURINOL

Xanthine oxidase inhibitor: ↓s uric acid synthesis.

Use: Px of **gout**, renal stones (urate or Ca^{2+} oxalate) and other ↑urate states (esp 2° to chemotherapy).

CI: acute gout: can worsen – don't start drug during attack (but don't stop drug if acute attack occurs during Rx).

Caution: R (↓dose), **L** (↓dose and monitor LFTs), **P/B**.

SE: GI upset, ☠ severe skin reactions ☠ (*stop drug if rash develops and allopurinol is implicated* – can reintroduce cautiously if mild reaction and no recurrence). Rarely, neuropathy (and many non-specific neurological symptoms), blood disorders, RF, hepatotoxicity, gynaecomastia, vasculitis.

Warn: report rashes, maintain good hydration.

Interactions: ↑s fx/toxicity of **azathioprine** (and possibly other cytotoxics, esp ciclosporin), chlorpropamide and theophyllines. Level ↓d by salicylates and probenecid. ↑rash with ampicillin and amox-icillin. **W** + .

Dose: initially 100 mg od po (↑if required to max of 900 mg/day in divided doses of up to 300 mg) after food. Usual dose 300 mg/day.
NB: ↓dose **in LF or RF**.
Initial Rx can ↑gout: give colchicine or NSAID (e.g. indometacin or diclofenac – *not aspirin*) Px until ≥1 month after urate normalised.

ALPHAGAN see Brimonidine; α-agonist eye drops for glaucoma.

ALTEPLASE ((recombinant) tissue-type plasminogen activator, rt-PA, TPA). Recombinant fibrinolytic.
Use: acute MI, acute massive PE (with haemodynamic instability). Acute ischaemic CVA w/in 3 h of onset (specialist use only).
CI/Caution/SE: See p. 215 for use in MI (for use in PE/CVA, see SPC). **L** (avoid if severe).
Dose: MI: total dose of 100 mg – regimen depends on time since onset of pain: *0–6 h*: 15 mg iv bolus, then 50 mg ivi over 30 min, then 35 mg ivi over 60 min; *6–12 h*: 10 mg iv bolus, then 50 mg ivi over 60 min, then four further 10 mg ivis, each over 30 min.
PE: 10 mg iv over 1–2 min then 90 mg ivi over 2 h.

> ☠ ↓doses if patient <65 kg; see SPC ☠. If MI concurrent unfractionated iv heparin needed for ≥24 h; see p. 215. Heparin also needed if giving for PE; see SPC.

ALUMINIUM HYDROXIDE

Antacid, PO_4-binding agent (↓s GI absorption).
Use: dyspepsia, ↑PO_4 (which can ↑risk of bone disease; esp good if secondary to RF, when ↑Ca^{2+} can occur dt ↑PTH, as other PO_4 binders often contain Ca^{2+}).
CI: ↓PO_4, porphyria.
SE: constipation*. Aluminium can accumulate in RF (esp on dialysis) ⇒ ↑risk of encephalopathy, dementia, osteomalacia.
Interactions: can ↓absorption of oral antibiotics (e.g. tetracyclines).
Dose: 1–2 (500-mg) tablets or 5–10 ml of 4% suspension prn (qds often sufficient). ↑doses to individual requirements, esp if for ↑PO_4. Also available as 475 mg capsules as Alucaps (contains ↓Na^+). Most effective taken with meals and at bedtime. Consider laxative Px*.

AMANTADINE

Weak DA agonist; ↑s release and ↓s reuptake of DA. Also antiviral properties; ↓s release of viral nucleic acid.

Use: Parkinson's disease and dyskinesias. Also used for Px of influenza A (if immunocompromised, vaccine CI or in exposed health workers).

CI: gastric ulcer (inc Hx of), epilepsy, **R** (if creatinine clearance < 15 ml/min), **P/B**.

Caution: confused or hallucinatory states **L/H/E**.

SE: confusion, hallucinations, leg oedema.

Warn: Can ↓skilled task performance (esp driving). Stop drug slowly*.

Interactions: memantine ↑risk of CNS toxicity, anticholinergics.

Dose: 100–400 mg daily[SPC/BNF]. NB: ↓dose in RF.

NB: stop slowly*: risk of withdrawal syndrome.

AMFEBUTAMONE see Bupropion; aid to smoking cessation.

AMILORIDE

K^+-sparing diuretic (weak): inhibits DCT Na^+ reabsorption and K^+ excretion.

Use: oedema (2° to HF, cirrhosis or ↑aldosterone), HTN (esp in conjunction with ↑K^+-wasting diuretics as combination preparations; see Co-amilofruse and Co-amilozide). *For advice on stepped HTN Mx see p. 182.*

CI: ↑K^+, Addison's, **R**.

Caution: DM (as risk of RF; monitor U&E), ↑risk of acidosis, ↓Na^+, **P/B/E**.

SE: ↑K^+, GI upset, headache, dry mouth, ↓BP (esp postural), ↓Na^+, rash, confusion. Rarely encephalopathy, hepatic/renal dysfunction.

Interactions: ↑s lithium levels. Can ↑nephrotoxicity of NSAIDs.

Dose: 2.5–20 mg od (or divide into bd doses).

> ☠ Beware if on other drugs that ↑K^+, e.g. spironolactone, triamterene, ACE-i, ARBs and ciclosporin. Don't give oral K^+ supplements inc dietary salt-substitute tablets ☠.

AMINOPHYLLINE

Methylxanthine bronchodilator: as theophylline but ↑H_2O solubility (is mixed w ethylenediamine) and ↓hypersensitivity.

L/R/H = Liver, Renal and Heart failure (full key see p. vii)

Use/CI/Caution/SE/Interactions: see Theophylline; also available iv for use in acute severe bronchospasm; see p. 247. ☠ NB: has many important interactions (dose adjustment may be needed) and can ⇒ arrhythmias (use cardiac monitor if giving iv)☠.

Monitor: serum levels at 6, 18 and 24 h after starting ivi. Also do levels initially if taking po.

Dose: po: MR preparation (**Phyllocontin continus**) ⇒ ↓SEs, has different doses at 225–450 mg bd (or 350–700 mg bd if Forte tablets – for smokers and others with short $t_{1/2}$). *If on a particular brand, ensure this is prescribed as they have different pharmacokinetics.* iv: load* with 5 mg/kg (usually = 250–500 mg) over ≥20 min, then 0.5 mg/kg/h ivi, then adjusted to keep plasma levels at 10–20 mg/l (= 55–110 micromol/l). If possible, contact pharmacy for dosing advice to consider interactions, obesity and liver/heart function.

☠If already taking maintenance po aminophylline/theophylline, omit loading dose* and check levels ASAP to guide dosing☠.

AMIODARONE

Class III antiarrhythmic: ↑s refractory period of conducting system; useful as has ↓negative inotropic fx than other drugs and can give when others ineffective/CI.

Use: tachyarrhythmias: esp paroxysmal SVT, AF, atrial flutter, nodal tachycardias, VT and VF. Also in CPR/periarrest arrhythmias.

CI: ↓HR (sinus), sinoatrial HB, SAN disease or severe conduction disturbance w/o pacemaker, Hx of thyroid disease/iodine sensitivity, **P/B**.

Caution: porphyria, ↓K⁺ (↑risk of torsades), **L/R/H/E**.

SE: *Acute:* N&V (dose-dependent), ↓HR/BP. *Chronic:* rarely but seriously ↑or ↓T4, interstitial lung disease (e.g. fibrosis, *but reversible if caught early*), **hepatotoxicity, conduction disturbances** (esp ↓HR). *Common:* **malaise, fatigue,** photosensitive skin (rarely 'grey-slate'), corneal deposits ± 'night glare' (reversible), tremor, sleep disorders. *Less commonly:* optic neuritis (rare but can ↓vision), peripheral neuropathy, blood disorders, hypersensitivity.

AMPICILLIN

Broad-spectrum penicillin for iv Use: has ↓GI absorption cf amox-icillin, which is preferred po.

Use: Meningitis (esp *Listeria*; see p. 179)[1], Px pre-operative or for endocarditis during invasive procedures if valve lesions/prostheses, respiratory tract/ENT infections (esp community-acquired pneumonia dt *Haemophilus influenzae* or *Streptococcus pneumoniae*), UTIs (not for blind Rx, as *Escherichia coli* often resistant).

CI: penicillin hypersensitivity (NB: cross-reactivity with cephalosporins possible).

Caution: EBV/CMV infections, ALL, CLL (all ↑risk of rash), **R**.

SE: rash (erythematous, maculopapular: often does not reflect true allergy) commoner in RF or crystal nephropathy **N&V&D** (rarely AAC), **hypersensitivity**, CNS/blood disorders.

Interactions: levels ↑by probenecid. ↑risk of rash with allopurinol. Can ↓fx of OCP (warn patient) and ↑levels of methotrexate.

Dose: Most indications 0.25–1 g qds po/im/iv[SPC/BNF] (meningitis 2 g 4-hrly ivi[1]). NB: ↓**dose in RF**.

ANTABUSE see Disulfiram; adjunct to alcohol withdrawal.

ANTACIDS see Alginates (e.g. Acidex, Gastrocote, Gaviscon or Peptac) or Co-magaldrox.

AQUEOUS CREAM Emulsifying ointment (phenoxyethanol in purified water). Topical cream used as emollient in dry skin conditions and as a soap-substitute.

▼ ARIPIPRAZOLE/ABILIFY

Atypical (third generation) antipsychotic; *partial* D_2 (and $5HT_{1A}$) agonist ⇒ ↓dopaminergic neuronal activity. Also potent $5HT_{2A}$ antagonist.

Use: schizophrenia, mania (Px and acute Rx).

CI: B.

Caution: cerebrovascular disease, Hx or ↑risk of seizures, family Hx of ↑QT **L/P/E**.

SE: EPSE (esp akathisia/restlessness, although generally ⇒ ↓EPSE than other antipsychotics), dizziness, sedation (or insomnia), blurred vision,

fatigue, headache, gastrointestinal upset, anxiety and ↑salivation. Rarely ↑HR, depression, orthostatic ↓BP. Very rarely skin/blood disorders, ↑QTc, DM, NMS, tardive dyskinesia, seizures and CVA.
Interactions: metab by P450 ∴ many; most importantly levels ↑ by itra-conazole, HIV protease/itra-conazole, HIV protease inhibitors and levels ↓ by carbamazepine, rifampicin, rifabutin, phenytoin, primodone, efavirenz, nevirapine and St John's wort.
Dose: 10–15 mg po od (max 30 mg/od); 5.25–15 (usually 9.75) mg im as single dose repeated after ≥2 h if required (max 3 injections/day or combined im/po dose of 30 mg/day). **NB:** ↓dose in elderly.

ARTHROTEC
Combination tablets of diclofenac with misoprostol (200 microgram/tablet) to ↓GI SEs (esp PU/bleeds).
CI/Caution/SE/Interactions: see Diclofenac and Misoprostol.
Dose: 50 mg bd/tds po or 75 mg bd (prescribed as dose of diclofenac).

ASACOL see Mesalazine: 'new' aminosalicylate for UC with ↓SEs.
Available po (3–6 tablets of 400 mg per day in divided doses), as suppositories (0.75–1.5 g daily in divided doses) or as foam enemas (1–2 g daily).

ASPIRIN
NSAID. Inhibits COX-1 and COX-2 ⇒ ↓PG synthesis (∴ anti-inflammatory and antipyrexial) and ↓thromboxane A_2 (∴ anti-Pt aggregation).
Use: mild to moderate pain/pyrexia[1], IHD and thromboembolic CVA Px[2] and acute Rx[3].
CI: < 16 years old, unless specifically indicated (can ⇒ Reye's syndrome), PU (active or PHx of), hypersensitivity to any NSAID, haemophilia, **R**(GFR < 10 ml/min)/**L**(if severe)/**B**.
Caution: asthma, any allergic disease*, dehydration, uncontrolled HTN, gout, G6PD deficiency, **L/R**(avoid if either severe)/**P/E**.
SE: GI irritation, bleeding (esp GI: ↑↑risk if also anticoagulated)**. Rarely hypersensitivity* (anaphylaxis, bronchospasm, skin reactions), AKI, hepatotoxicity, ototoxic in OD.

Interactions: ↑GI bleeding with anticoagulants**, other NSAIDs (avoid), SSRIs & venlafaxine. **W** + Can ⇒ ↑levels of methotrexate, ↑fx anticonvulsants & ↓fx spironolactone.
Dose: 300–900 mg 4–6-hrly (max 4 g/day)[1], 75 mg od[2], 300 mg stat[3].

> Stop 7 days before surgery if significant bleeding is expected. If cardiac surgery or patient has ACS, consider continuing.

ATENOLOL

β-blocker: (mildly) cardioselective* ($β_1 > β_2$), ↑H_2O solubility ∴ ↓central fx** and ↑renal excretion***.
Use: HTN[1] (*for advice on stepped HTN Mx see p. 182*), angina[2], MI (w/in 12 h as early intervention)[3], arrhythmias[4].
CI/Caution/SE/Interactions: see Propranolol ⇒ ↓bronchospasm* (but avoid in all asthma/only use in COPD if no other choice) and ↓sleep disturbance/nightmares**.
Dose: 25–50 mg od po[1]; 100 mg od po[2]; 5 mg iv over 5 min then 50 mg po 15 min later then start 50 mg bd 12 h later[3]; 50–100 mg od po[4] (for iv doses see SPC/BNF). **NB: consider ↓dose in RF***.**

ATORVASTATIN/LIPITOR

H MG-CoA reductase inhibitor.
Use/CI/Caution/SE: see Simvastatin.
Interactions: ↑risk of myopathy with ☠fibrates☠, daptomycin, ciclosporin, nicotinic acid, itra-/posa-conazole. Levels ↑by clari-/telithromycin.
Dose: initially 10 mg nocte (↑if necessary, at intervals ≥4 wks, to max 80 mg). Post ACS dose 80 mg daily.

iv ATROPINE (SULPHATE)

Muscarinic antagonist: blocks vagal SAN and AVN stimulation, bronchodilates and ↓s oropharyngeal secretions.
Use: severe ↓HR (see algorithm on inside front cover) or HB[1], CPR[2] (see ALS universal algorithm on inside back cover), organophosphate/anticholinesterase* OD/poisoning[3] and specialist anaesthetic uses.

CI: (*don't apply if life-threatening condition/CPR!*): glaucoma (angle closure), MG (*unless anticholinesterase overdosage*, when atropine is indicated*), paralytic ileus, pyloric stenosis, bladder neck obstruction (e.g. ↑prostate).

Caution: Down's syndrome, gastro-oesophageal reflux, diarrhoea, UC, acute MI, HTN, ↑HR (esp 2° to ↑T_4, cardiac insufficiency or surgery), pyrexia, P/B/E.

SE: transient ↓HR (followed by ↑HR, palpitations, arrhythmias), **antimuscarinic fx** (see p. 233), N&V, confusion (esp in elderly), dizziness.

Dose: 0.3–1.0 mg iv[1]; 3 mg iv[2] (*if no iv/intraosseous access, give 6 mg with 10 ml saline via endotracheal tube*); 1–2 mg im/iv every 10–30 min[3] (every 5 min in severe cases) to max 100 mg in 1st 24 h, until symptomatic response (skin flushes and dries, pupils dilate, HR↑s).

ATROVENT see Ipratropium; bronchodilator for COPD/asthma.

AUGMENTIN see Co-amoxiclav (amoxicillin + clavulanic acid) 375 or 625 mg tds po (1.2 g tds iv).

AZATHIOPRINE

Antiproliferative immunosuppressant: inhibits purine-salvage p'ways; prodrug for 6-mercaptopurine.

Use: prevention of transplant rejection, autoimmune disease (esp as steroid-sparing agent, but also maintenance Rx for SLE/vasculitis).

CI: hypersensitivity (to azathioprine *or mercaptopurine*), P/B.

Caution: L/R/E.

SE: **myelosuppression** (dose-dependent, ⇒ ↑infections, esp HZV), **hepatotoxicity, hypersensitivity reactions** (inc interstitial nephritis: *stop drug!*), N&V&D (esp initially), pancreatitis. Rarely cholestasis, alopecia, pneumonitis, risk of neoplasia, hepatic veno-occlusion.

Warn: immediately report infections or unexpected bruising/ bleeding.

Monitor: FBC (initially ≥wkly ↓ing to ≥3-monthly), LFTs, U&Es.

Interactions: fx ↑ by **allopurinol**, ACE-i, ARBs, trimethoprim (and septrin). fx ↓ by rifampicin. W−.

Caution: cardiovascular disease, PU, porphyria, Raynaud's disease, serious Ψ disorders (esp psychosis), **P/B**.

SE: GI upset, postural ↓BP (esp initially and if ↑alcohol intake), **behavioural Δs** (confusional states, Ψ disorders), ↑sleep (sudden onset/daytime). Rarely but seriously **fibrosis***: pulmonary**, cardiac, retroperitoneal*** (can ⇒ AKI).

Warn: of ↑sleep. Report persistent cough** or chest/abdo pain.

Monitor: ESR*, U&Es***, CXR**; pituitary size and visual fields (pregnancy and[1])**.

Interactions: levels ↑by ery-/clari-thromycin and octreotide.

Dose: 1–30 mg/day[SPC/BNF]. NB: consider ↓dose in LF.

BUCCASTEM Prochlorperazine (antiemetic) buccal tablets: absorbed rapidly from under top lip ∴ don't need to be swallowed and retained in stomach for absorption if N&V.

Caution: L.

Dose: 3–6 mg bd.

▼ BUDESONIDE

Inh corticosteroid for asthma[1]; similar to beclometasone but stronger (approximately double the strength per microgram). Also available po or as enemas for IBD[2] (see BNF).

Caution: L.

Dose: 200–800 microgram bd inh (aerosol or powder) or 1–2 mg bd neb[1].

BUMETANIDE

Loop diuretic: inhibits Na^+/K^+ pump in ascending loop of Henle.

Use/CI/Caution/SE/Monitor/Interactions: as furosemide; also headaches, gynaecomastia and at ↑doses can ⇒ myalgia.

Dose: 1 mg mane po (500 microgram may suffice in elderly), ↑ing if required (5 mg/24 h usually sufficient; ↑by adding a lunchtime dose, then ↑ing each dose). 1–2 mg im/iv (repeat after 20 min if required). 2–5 mg ivi over 30–60 min.

NB: give iv in severe oedema; bowel oedema ⇒ ↓po absorption.

BUPROPION (= AMFEBUTAMONE)/ZYBAN

NA and to lesser extent DA reuptake inhibitor (NDRI) developed as antidepressant, but also ↑s success of giving up smoking.

Use: (adjunct to) smoking cessation[NICE].

CI: CNS tumour, acute alcohol/benzodiazepine withdrawal, Hx of seizures*, eating disorders, bipolar disorder, **L** (if severe cirrhosis)/**P/B**.

Caution: if ↑risk of seizures*: alcohol abuse, Hx of head trauma and DM, **R/E**.

SE: seizures*, **insomnia** (and other CNS reactions, e.g. anxiety, agitation, depression, fever, headaches, tremor, dizziness). Also ↑HR, AV block, ↑or ↓BP**, chest pain, hypersensitivity (inc severe skin reactions), GI upset, ↑Wt, mild antimuscarinic fx (esp **dry mouth**; see p. 233 for others).

Monitor: BP**.

Interactions: ↓P450 ∴ many interactions, but importantly **CNS drugs**, esp if ↓seizure threshold*, e.g. antidepressants (☠ MAOIs; avoid together, including <2 wks after MAOI☠), antimalarials, antipsychotics (esp risperidone), quinolones, sedating antihistamines, systemic corticosteroids, theophyllines, tramadol. Ritonavir ⇒ ↓plasma level of bupropion.

Dose: 150 mg od for 6 days then 150 mg bd for max 9 wks (↓dose if elderly or ↑seizure risk[SPC/BNF]). Start 1–2 wks before target date of stopping smoking. **NB: max 150 mg/day in LF or RF.**

BURINEX Bumetanide 1-mg tablets.

BUSCOPAN see Hyoscine butylbromide; GI antispasmodic.

CACIT see Calcium carbonate.

CACIT D3 Calcium carbonate + low dose vitamin D_3.
Use: Px of vitamin D deficiency.
Caution: **L**.
Dose: 1 tablet od (= 12.5 mmol Ca^{2+} + 11 microgram cholecalciferol).

CALCICHEW see Calcium carbonate.

SE: GI upset (esp N&D, but also AAC), **allergy** (anaphylaxis, fever, arthralgia, skin reactions (inc severe)), **AKI, interstitial nephritis** (reversible), hepatic dysfunction, blood disorders, CNS disturbance (inc headache).

Interactions: levels ↑by probenecid, mild **W** + .

Dose: 250 mg tds po (500 mg tds in severe infections; max 4 g/day). NB: ↓dose in RF.

Cephalosporins can ⇒ false-positive Coombs' and urine glucose tests.

CEFALEXIN

Oral 1st-generation cephalosporin.

Use/CI/Caution/SE/Interactions: see Cefaclor and **AAC warning**.

Dose: 250 mg qds or 500 mg bd/tds po (↑in severe infections to max 1.5 g qds). For Px of UTI, give 125 mg po nocte. NB: ↓dose in RF.

CEFOTAXIME

Parenteral 3rd-generation cephalosporin. Good Gram-neg activity, except *Pseudomonas*.

Use: severe infections, esp meningitis and typhoid, UTI, pyelone-phritis, soft-tissue infections, gonorrhoea.

CI/Caution/SE/Interactions: see Cefaclor and **AAC warning**, but can also rarely ⇒ arrhythmias if given as rapid iv injection.

Dose: 1 g bd im/iv/ivi (↑ing to max of 3 g qds if needed). NB: ↓dose in RF.

CEFRADINE

Oral or parenteral 1st-generation cephalosporin.

Use: as cefaclor.

CI/Caution/SE/Interactions: see Cefaclor and **AAC warning**.

Dose: po: 250–500 mg qds or 0.5–1 g bd (max 1 g qds). NB: ↓dose in RF.

CEFTAZIDIME

Parenteral 3rd-generation cephalosporin: good against *Pseudomonas*.

Use: see Cefotaxime (often reserved for ITU setting).

CI/Caution/SE/Interactions: see Cefaclor and **AAC warning**.
Dose: 1 g tds im/iv/ivi, ↑ing (with care in elderly) to 2 g tds or 3 g bd iv (not im, where max single dose is 1 g) if life-threatening, e.g. meningitis, immunocompromised. **NB: ↓dose in RF.**

CEFTRIAXONE

Parenteral 3rd-generation cephalosporin.
Use: as cefotaxime, plus pre-operative Px[1].
CI/Caution/SE/Interactions: as Cefaclor and **AAC warning**, plus **L** (if coexistent RF), **R** (if severe), caution if dehydrated, young or immobile (can precipitate in urine or gallbladder). Rarely ⇒ pancreatitis and ↑PT.
Dose: 1 g od im/iv/ivi (max 4 g/day); 1–2 g im/iv/ivi at induction[1].
NB: ↓dose in RF.

Max im dose = 1 g per site; if total >1 g, give at divided sites.

CEFUROXIME

Parenteral and oral 2nd-generation cephalosporin: good for some Gram-negative infections (*H. influenzae*, *N. gonorrhoeae*) and better than 3rd-generation cephalosporins for Gram-positive infections (esp *S. aureus*).
Use: po: respiratory infections[1], UTIs[2], pyelonephritis[3]; **iv:** severe infections[4], pre-operative Px[5].
CI/Caution/SE/Interactions: see Cefaclor and **AAC warning**.
Dose: 250–500 mg bd po[1]; 125 mg bd po[2]; 250 mg bd po[3]; 750 mg tds/qds iv/im[4] (1.5 g tds/qds iv in very severe infections and 3 g tds if meningitis); 1.5 g iv at induction (+750 mg iv/im tds for 24 h if high-risk procedure)[5]. **NB: ↓dose in RF.**

CELECOXIB/CELEBREX

NSAID which selectively inhibits COX-2 ∴ ↓GI SEs (COX-1 mediated).
Use: osteoarthritis/RA[NICE], ankylosing spondylitis. Beneficial GI fx (↓bleeding) lost if on aspirin ∴ don't use together.

Interactions: May ↑sedation caused by alcohol and sedative medications. May ↑hypotension caused by other medications, fx ↑d by TCAs (esp antimuscarinic fx), lithium (esp extrapyramidal fx ± neurotoxicity), ritonavir, cimetidine and β-blockers (esp arrhythmias with sotalol; propranolol fx also ↑d by chlorpromazine). ↑risk of CNS toxicity with sibutramine. Avoid artemether/lumefantrine and drugs that ↑QTc or risk of ventricular arrhythmias (e.g. disopyramide, moxifloxacin).
Dose: 25–300 mg tds po[SPC/BNF]; 25–50 mg tds/qds im (painful, and may ⇒ ↓BP/↑HR). **NB: ↓dose in elderly (approx 1/3–1/2 adult dose but 10 mg od po may suffice) or if severe RF.**

CICLESONIDE/ALVESCO

Inh corticosteroid for asthma, similar to beclomethasone but od.
Caution: L.
Dose: 80–160 microgram od inh (aerosol).

CICLOSPORIN

Calcineurin inhibitor: ⇒ ↓IL-2-mediated LØ proliferation.
Use: immunosuppression (esp nephrotic syndrome and post-transplant), atopic dermatitis, psoriasis, RA.
CI: *only apply if given for nephrotic syndrome*: uncontrolled infection or HTN, malignancy. Avoid co-treatment with sirolimus.
Caution: HTN, ↑urate, porphyria, drugs that ↑K^+, **L/R/P/B/E.**
SE: nephrotoxicity and **tremor** (both dose-related), ↑BP, hepatotoxicity, GI upset, biochemical Δs (↑K^+, ↑urate/gout, ↓Mg^{2+}, ↑cholesterol, ↑glucose), pancreatitis. Rarely neuromuscular symptoms, HUS, neoplasms (esp lymphoma), BIH, encephalopathy, demyelination (esp if liver transplant).
Warn: hypertrichosis, gingival hypertrophy, avoid XS sun exposure (photosensitivity); burning sensation in hands and feet.
Monitor: levels, LFTs, U&Es, Mg^{2+}, lipids, BP.
Interactions: metab by **P450,** ∴ many, particularly antibacterials and antifungals[SPC/BNF] (cephalosporins and penicillins OK). Levels esp ↓by phenytoin, carbamazepine, phenobarbital, St John's wort, rifampicin, orlistat, ticlopidine and octreotide. Levels esp ↑by ery-/clari-thromycin,

keto-/flu-/itra-conazole, protease inhibitors, diltiazem, nicardipine, verapamil, metoclopramide, amiodarone, allopurinol, danazol, ursodeoxycholic acid, corticosteroids and OCP. Can ↑levels of digoxin and diclofenac. Nephrotoxic and myotoxic drugs can become more so.
Dose: specialist use[SPC/BNF]. Must prescribe by brand name (**Neoral, Sandimmun** or **SangCya**) as have different bioavailabilities and changing brands can ∴ ↓immunosuppression or ↑toxicity. **NB: dose adjustment needed if LF or RF.**

> 💀 Check all new drugs for interactions before prescribing if on ciclosporin: ↑d levels ⇒ toxicity; ↓d levels may ⇒ rejection 💀.

CIMETIDINE

As ranitidine, but ↑↑interactions (↓**P450** and **W**+) and ↑gynaecomastia ∴ prescribed rarely. **Dose:** 400 mg bd (can ↑to 4-hrly[SPC/BNF]). NB: ↓**dose if LF or RF.**

CIPROFLOXACIN

(Fluoro)quinolone antibiotic: inhibits DNA gyrase; 'cidal' with broad spectrum, but particularly good for Gram-negative infections.
Use: GI infections[1] (esp salmonella, shigella, campylobacter), respiratory infections (non-pneumococcal pneumonias[2], esp *Pseudomonas*). Also GU infections (esp UTIs[3], acute uncomplicated cystitis in women[4], gonorrhoea[5]), 1st-line initial Rx of anthrax.
CI: hypersensitivity to any quinolone, **P/B**.
Caution: seizures (inc Hx of, or predisposition to), MG (can worsen), G6PD deficiency, children/adolescents (theoretical risk of arthropathy), avoid ↑urine pH or dehydration*, **R**.
SE: GI upset (esp N&D, sometimes AAC), pancreatitis, neuro-Ψ fx (esp confusion, **seizures**; also headache, dizziness, hallucinations, sleep and mood Δs), **tendinitis** ± **rupture** (esp if elderly or taking steroids), chest pain, oedema, **hypersensitivity** (rash, pruritis, fever). Rarely hepatotoxicity, RF/interstitial nephritis, crystalluria*, blood disorders, ↑glucose, skin reactions (inc photosensitivity**, SJS, TEN).
Warn: avoid UV light**, avoid ingesting Fe- and Zn-containing products (e.g. antacids***). May impair skilled tasks/driving.

Interactions: ↑s levels of theophyllines; NSAIDs ⇒ ↑risk of seizures; ↑s nephrotoxicity of ciclosporin; $FeSO_4$ and antacids*** ⇒ ↓ciprofloxacin absorption (give 2 h before or 6 h after ciprofloxacin), **W +** .

Dose: 250–750 mg bd po, 100–400 mg bd ivi (each dose over 1 h) according to indication[SPC/BNF] (100 mg bd po for 3 days for cystitis); 500 mg po single dose[4]; 100 mg iv single dose[5]. **NB: ↓dose if severe RF.**

☠ Stop if tendinitis, severe neuro-Ψ fx or hypersensitivity ☠ .

CITALOPRAM/CIPRAMIL

SSRI antidepressant.

Use: depression[1] (and panic disorder). Useful if polypharmacy, as ↓interactions and ↓cardio-/hepato-toxicity cf other SSRIs (see p. 197).

CI/Caution/SE/Warn: as fluoxetine, but ↑risk of withdrawal syndrome if stopped abruptly. Can also ↑QT_c (dose dependent); CI if ↑QT_c (or congenital ↑QT_c syndrome or taking other drugs that can ↑QT_c) and caution if ↑risk torsades de pointes (e.g. congestive HF, recent MI, bradyarrhythmias, predisposition to ↓K^+ or ↓Mg^{2+} dt concomitant illness or medicines).

Interaction: ☠ Never give with, or <2 wks after, MAOIs ☠ .

Dose: 20 mg od[1] ↑ing if necessary to max 40 mg (max 20 mg **if elderly or LF**).

CITRAMAG see Bowel preparations

CI: R (if severe).

Caution: risk of ↑Mg^{2+} in RF.

Dose: 1 sachet at 8 am and 3 pm the day before GI surgery or Ix.

CLARITHROMYCIN

Macrolide antibiotic: binds 50S ribosome.

Use: as erythromycin; see p. 172), part of triple therapy for *H. pylori* (see p. 177).

CI/Caution/SE/Interactions: as erythromycin, but ⇒ ↓GI SEs.

Dose: 250–500 mg bd po or 500 mg bd iv. **NB: ↓dose if RF.**

CLEXANE see Enoxaparin; low-molecular-weight heparin.

CLINDAMYCIN

Antibiotic; same action (but different structure and ∴ class) as clarithromycin; good against staphylococci, streptococci and anaerobes (esp bacteroides); penetrates bone well.
Use: cellulitis, osteomyelitis, intra-abdominal sepsis, endocarditis Px, falciparum malaria. Alternative to penicillin in case of allergy. *Use limited due to SEs (esp AAC).*
CI: diarrhoea.
Caution: GI disease, porphyria, atopy, **L/R/P/B**.
SE: GI upset (often ⇒ **AAC**), hepatotoxicity, blood disorders, local reactions at injection site, arthralgia, myalgia, hypersensitivity.
Monitor: U&Es, LFTs.
Interactions: ↑s fx of neuromuscular blocking agents.
Dose: 150–450 mg qds po; 0.6–4.8 g daily in divided doses im/ivi (doses >600 mg must be as ivi), max single dose iv is 1.2 g.

☠ Stop drug if diarrhoea develops: AAC common and potentially very severe.

CLOBETASOL PROPIONATE 0.05% CREAM OR OINTMENT/DERMOVATE

Very-potent-strength topical corticosteroid.
Use: short-term Rx of severe inflammatory skin conditions (esp discoid lupus, lichen simplex and palmar plantar psoriasis).
CI: untreated infection, rosacea, acne.
SE: skin atrophy, worsening of infections, acne (↑SEs cf less potent topical steroids).
Dose: apply thinly od/bd, usually under specialist supervision.

CLOBETASONE BUTYRATE 0.05% CREAM OR OINTMENT/EUMOVATE

Moderately-potent-strength topical corticosteroid.
Use: inflammatory skin conditions, esp eczema.
CI: untreated infection, rosacea, acne.
SE: skin atrophy, worsening of infections, acne.
Dose: apply thinly od/bd.

CLONAZEPAM

Benzodiazepine; long-acting (see p. 229)

Use: epilepsy (all forms[1] inc status epilepticus[2]). Not licensed, but often used, for Ψ disorders[3] (esp psychosis and mania).

CI/Caution/SE/Warn/Interactions: see Diazepam.

Dose: 0.5–1 mg ↑ing according to response to max 20 mg/day[1/3] in divided doses; 1 mg iv (over ≥2 min) or as ivi[2].

CLOPIDOGREL/PLAVIX

Antiplatelet agent: ADP receptor antagonist. ↑antiplatelet fx cf aspirin (but also ↑SEs).

Use: Px of atherothrombotic events if STEMI or NSTEMI (for 12 months in combination with aspirin, aspirin continued indefinitely), MI (within 'a few' to 35 days), ischaemic CVA (within 7 days to 6 months) or peripheral arterial disease. For use in ACS (see p. 240).

CI: active bleeding, **L** (if severe – otherwise caution), **B**.

Caution: ↑bleeding risk; trauma, surgery, drugs that ↑bleeding risk (*not recommended with* warfarin), **R/P**.

SE: haemorrhage (esp GI or intracranial), **GI upset**, PU, pancreatitis, headache, fatigue, dizziness, paraesthesia, rash/pruritus, hepatobiliary/respiratory/blood disorders (↓NØ, ↑EØ, very rarely, TTP).

Monitor: FBC and for signs of occult bleeding (esp after invasive procedures).

Dose: 75 mg od. If not already on clopidogrel, usually load with 300 mg for ACS then 75 mg od starting next day. If pre-PCI, load with 300–600 mg usually on morning of procedure.

> Stop 7 days before operations if antiplatelet fx not wanted (e.g. major surgery); discuss with surgeons doing operation.

CLOTRIMAZOLE/CANESTEN

Imidazole antifungal (topical).

Use: external candida infections (esp vaginal thrush).

Caution: can damage condoms and diaphragms.

Dose: 2–3 applications/day of 1% cream, continuing for 14 days after lesion healed. Also available as powder/solution/spray for hairy areas, as pessary, and in 2% strength.

CLOZAPINE

Atypical antipsychotic: blocks dopamine ($D_4 > D_1 > D_{2 \text{ and } 3}$) and $5HT_{2A}$ receptors. Also mild blockade of muscarinic and adrenergic receptors.

Use: schizophrenia, but only if resistant or intolerant (e.g. severe extrapyramidal fx) to other antipsychotics[NICE].

CI: severe cardiac disorders (inc Hx of circulatory collapse, myocarditis, cardiomyopathy), coma/severe CNS depression, alcoholic/toxic psychosis, drug intoxication, Hx of agranulocytosis or ↓NØ, bone marrow disorders, paralytic ileus, uncontrolled epilepsy, **R/H** (if severe, otherwise caution), **L** (inc active liver disease), **B**.

Caution: Hx of epilepsy, cardiovascular disease, ↑prostate, glaucoma (angle-closure), **P/E**.

SE: as olanzapine, but also can ⇒ ↓NØ* (3% of patients) and ☠ **agranulocytosis** ☠ (1%). Also commonly ⇒ ↑**salivation** (Rx with hyoscine hydrobromide), ↓**BP** (esp during initial titration), **constipation** (can ⇒ ileus/obstruction: have low threshold for giving laxatives), ↑Wt, sedation. Less commonly seizures, urinary incontinence, priapism, **myocarditis/cardiomyopathy** (*stop immediately!*), ↑HR, arrhythmias, hyperglycaemia, N&V, ↑BP, delirium, RF, ↓Pt. Rarely hepatic dysfunction (*stop immediately!*), ↑TG, neuroleptic malignant syndrome.

Monitor: FBC*, BP (esp during start of Rx), serum levels (pre-dose) and cardiac function (get baseline ECG/watch for persistent ↑HR).

Warn: to report symptoms of infection, e.g. fever, sore throat.

Interactions: as chlorpromazine, plus care with all drugs that constipate, ↑QT threshold or ↓leucopoiesis (e.g. cytotoxics, sulphonamides/co-trimoxazole, chloramphenicol, penicillamine, carbamazepine, phenothiazines, esp depots). Caffeine, risperidone, SSRIs, cimetidine and erythromycin ↑clozapine levels. Smoking, carbamazepine and phenytoin ↓clozapine levels.

Dose: initially 12.5 mg nocte, ↑ing to 200–450 mg/day[SPC/BNF] usually given bd (max 900 mg/day). ↓doses if elderly.

If >2 days' doses missed, restart at 12.5 mg od and ↑gradually.

> **Monitoring:** primarily to avoid fatal agranulocytosis, is done by the manufacturers: in the UK Clozaril Patient Monitoring Service (tel: 0845 7698269), Denzapine Monitoring Service (tel: 0845 0090110) or Zaponex Treatment Access System (tel: 0207 3655842). Register and then authorise/monitor baseline and subsequent FBCs* and serum levels*. *These are very useful resources for all clozapine questions.*

CO-AMILOFRUSE

Diuretic combination preparation for oedema that keeps K^+ stable: amiloride (K^+-sparing) + furosemide (K^+-wasting) in 3 strengths of tablet as 2.5/20, 5/40 and 10/80 (reflecting amiloride mg/furosemide mg).
Monitor: BP, U&Es.
Dose: 1 tablet mane (NB: *specify strength!*).

CO-AMILOZIDE

Diuretic combination preparation for HTN (*for advice on stepped HTN Mx see p. 182*), CCF and oedema. Keeps K^+ stable: amiloride (K^+-sparing) + hydrochlorothiazide (K^+-wasting) in 2 strengths of tablet as 2.5/25 and 5/50 (reflecting amiloride mg/hydrochlorothiazide mg).
Caution: crystalluria esp if ↑dose or RF.
Monitor: BP, U&Es.
Dose: 1/2–4 tablets daily, according to tablet strength and indication[SPC/BNF].

CO-AMOXICLAV/AUGMENTIN

Combination of amoxicillin + clavulanic acid (β-lactamase inhibitor) to overcome resistance.
Use: UTIs, respiratory/skin/soft-tissue (plus many other) infections. Reserve for when β-lactamase-producing strains known/strongly suspected or other Rx has failed.

CI/Caution/SE/Interactions: as ampicillin, plus caution if antic-oagulated, **L** (↑risk of cholestasis), **P**.
Dose: as amoxicillin Dose: 250 mg tds po (500 mg tds po if severe); 1 g tds/qds iv/ivi. Non-proprietary and as **Augmentin**. NB: ↓dose if LF.

CO-BENELDOPA/MADOPAR

L-dopa + benserazide (peripheral dopa-decarboxylase inhibitor).
Use: Parkinsonism.
CI/Caution/SE/Warn/Interactions: see Levodopa.
Dose: (*expressed as levodopa only*) initially 50 mg tds/qds, ↑ing total dose and number of doses, according to response, to usual maintenance of 400–800 mg/day (↓in elderly). Available in dispersible form.

CO-CARELDOPA/SINEMET

L-dopa + carbidopa (peripheral dopa-decarboxylase inhibitor).
Use: Parkinsonism.
CI/Caution/SE/Warn/Interactions: see Levodopa.
Dose: (*expressed as levodopa only*) initially 50–100 mg tds, ↑ing total dose and number of doses, according to response, to usual maintenance of 400–800 mg/day (↓in elderly). Available in dispersible form.

CO-CODAMOL (8/500) = codeine 8 mg + paracetamol 500 mg per tablet.

Use/CI/Caution/SE/Interactions: see Paracetamol and Codeine.
Warning: prescribe by dose as also available as 15/500 and 30/500.
Dose: 2 tablets qds prn. NB: ↓dose if LF, RF or elderly.

CO-DANTHRAMER see Dantron; stimulant laxative.
Dose: 1–2 capsules or 5–10 ml suspension nocte (available in regular and strong formulations).

CO-DANTHRUSATE see Dantron; stimulant laxative.
Dose: 1–3 capsules or 5–15 ml suspension nocte.

CODEINE (PHOSPHATE)

Weak opiate analgesic. Mainly metabolised to morphine.

Use: mild/moderate pain, diarrhoea, anti-tussive.

CI: acute respiratory depression, risk of ileus, ↑ICP/head injury/coma.

Caution: all other conditions where morphine is either contra-indicated or cautioned.

SE: as morphine, but milder. **Constipation** is the major problem: dose and length of Rx-dependent; anticipate this and give laxative Px as appropriate, esp in elderly. Also sedation, esp if LF.

Interactions: ☠ MAOIs: don't give within 2 weeks of ☠. As morphine, but does not interact with baclofen, gabapentin and ritonavir.

Dose: 30–60 mg up to 4-hrly po/im (max 240 mg/24 h). Genetic ultrarapid metabolisers (3% of Europeans, 8% of Americans, 40% of North Africans) risk serious toxicity & poor metabolisers obtain little analgesia. Watch closely when initiating & adjust dose/change drug accordingly. **NB:** ↓dose if LF, RF or elderly.

CO-DYDRAMOL Dihydrocodeine 10/20/30 mg + paracetamol 500 mg per tablet (10/500, 20/500, 30/500).

Dose: 1–2 tablets 4–6 hrly, max qds po. Usually prescribed 2 tablets qds (prn). **NB:** ↓dose if LF, RF or elderly.

COLCHICINE

Anti-gout: binds to tubulin of leucocytes and stops their migration to uric acid deposits ∴ ⇒ ↓inflammation. NB: slow action (needs >6 h to work).

Use: gout: Rx of acute attacks or Px when starting allopurinol* (which can initially ↑symptoms) or awaiting other drugs to work.

CI: blood dyscrasias, **P**

Caution: GI diseases, **L/H/R/B/E**.

SE: GI upset (N&V&D and **abdominal pain** – all common and dose-related). Rarely GI haemorrhage, hypersensitivity, renal/hepatic impairment, peripheral neuritis, myopathy, alopecia, ↓spermatogenesis (reversible), blood disorders (if prolonged Rx).

Interactions: ↑s nephro-/myo-toxicity of ciclosporin and myopathy of simvastatin. fx ↓by thiazide diuretics. Toxicity ↑by erythromycin and tolbutamide.

Dose: 0.5 mg bd/qds for 7 days (start ASAP after symptom onset). More aggressive loading regimens exist[SPC/BNF] but ⇒ ↑GI upset w/o significant ↑in response. Continue 0.5 mg bd when starting allopurinol*. NB: ↓dose if RF.

COLESTYRAMINE

Anion exchange resin. Binds bile acids in gut preventing reabsorption; ⇒ ↑hepatic cholesterol ⇒ bile acids; ⇒ ↑hepatic LDL receptors ⇒ ↑LDL cholesterol plasma clearance.

Use: pruritus (2° to PBC or partial biliary obstruction)[1], diarrhoeal disorders[2]. *If diet and other measures insufficient*: hyperlipidaemia[3] (esp type IIa), Px of IHD[4], 1° hypercholesterolaemia[5].

CI: ineffective in complete biliary obstruction.

Caution: Risk of ↓vitamins. Sachets contain sucrose or aspartame. DM. **P/B**.

SE: ↓Vits A/D/K, ↑bleeding risk, taste Δ, GI upset/obstruction, ↑Cl⁻ acidosis.

Warn: take other drugs >1 h before or > 4–6 h after colestyramine*.

Monitor: for vitamin deficiency (and INR if on warfarin).

Interactions: delay or ↓drug absorption* inc digoxin, tetracycline, chlorothiazide, thyroxine. **W + or W–**.

Dose: initially 4 g od, ↑ing if required by 4 g/wk to 8 g/day[1] (max 36 g/day[2,3,4,5])

NB: take with ≥150 ml suitable liquid/4 g sachet.

CO-MAGALDROX antacid (AlOH + MgOH).

Dose: 10–20 ml 20–60 min after meals, and at bedtime or prn.

COMBIVENT Compound bronchodilator (salbutamol + ipratropium bromide).

Dose: 2.5 ml (one vial: ipratropium 500 microgram + salbutamol 2.5 mg) tds/qds neb[SPC/BNF].

CORSODYL Chlorhexidine mouthwash for Rx/Px of mouth infections (inc MRSA eradication); see local infection protocol.

CO-TRIAMTERZIDE

Diuretic for HTN[1] (*for advice on stepped HTN Mx see p. 182*), or oedema[2]: triamterene ($\uparrow$s K$^+$) combined with hydrochlorothiazide ($\downarrow$s K$^+$) to keep K$^+$ stable.

Monitor: BP, U&Es.

Dose: initially 1 tablet[1] (or 2 tablets[2]) mane of 50/25 strength (= 50 mg triamterene + 25 mg hydrochlorothiazide), $\uparrow$ing if necessary to max of 4 tablets/day.

CO-TRIMOXAZOLE/SEPTRIN

Antibiotic combination preparation: 5 to 1 mixture of sulfamethoxazole (a sulphonamide) + trimethoprim $\Rightarrow$ synergistic action.

Use: PCP; other uses limited due to SEs (also rarely used for toxoplasmosis and nocardiosis).

CI: porphyria, **L/R** (if either severe, otherwise caution).

Caution: blood disorders, asthma, G6PD deficiency, risk factors for $\downarrow$folate **P/B/E**.

SE: skin reactions (inc SJS, TEN), blood disorders ($\downarrow$NØ, $\downarrow$Pt, $\downarrow$Glucose, BM suppression, agranulocytosis) relatively common, esp in elderly. Also N&V&D (inc AAC), nephrotoxicity, hepatotoxicity, hypersensitivity, anorexia, abdo pain, glossitis, stomatitis, pancreatitis, arthralgia, myalgia, SLE, pulmonary infiltrates, seizures, ataxia, myocarditis.

Interactions: $\uparrow$s phenytoin levels. $\uparrow$s risk of arrhythmias with amiodarone, crystalluria with methenamine, antifolate fx with pyrimethamine, agranulocytosis with clozapine and toxicity with ciclosporin, azathioprine, mercaptopurine and methotrexate. **W +**.

Dose: PCP Rx: 120 mg/kg/day po/ivi in 2–4 divided doses (PCP Px 480–960 mg od po). **NB:** $\downarrow$**dose if RF**.

> ☠ Stop immediately if rash or blood disorder occurs ☠.

CYCLIZINE

Antihistamine antiemetic.

Use: N&V Rx/Px (esp 2° to iv/im opioids, but not 1st choice in angina/MI/LVF*), vertigo, motion sickness, labyrinthine disorders.

CI/Caution/SE/Warn: as chlorphenamine, but also avoid in severe HF* (may undo haemodynamic benefits of opioids). Antimuscarinic fx (see p. 233) are most prominent SEs.

Dose: 50 mg po/im/iv tds.

CYCLOPENTOLATE 0.5%/1% EYE DROPS/MYDRILATE

For pupil dilation (for pain relief and prevention of complications in uveitis). Also cycloplegic (paralyses accommodation); useful for refracting children.

SE: blurred vision.

Dose: 1 drop (tds for prolonged use). 30 min to work, lasts several hours.

CYCLOPHOSPHAMIDE

Cytotoxic[1] and immunosuppressant[2]: alkylating agent (cross-links DNA bases, ↓ing replication).

Use: cancer[1], autoimmune diseases[2]: esp vasculitis (inc rheumatoid arthritis, ANCA-associated vasculitis and SLE (esp if renal/cerebral involvement)), systemic sclerosis, Wegener's, nephrotic syndrome in children.

CI: haemorrhagic cystitis, **P/B**.

Caution: BM suppression, severe infections, **L/R**.

SE: GI upset, **alopecia** (reversible). Others rare but important: hepatotoxicity, blood disorders, malignancy (esp acute myeloid leukaemia), ↓**fertility** (can be permanent), cardiac toxicity, pulmonary fibrosis (at high doses), **haemorrhagic cystitis** (only if given **iv**: ensure good hydration, give 'mesna' as Px; can occur months after Rx).

Warn: ↓fertility may be permanent (bank sperm if possible) – need to counsel and obtain consent regarding this before giving.

Monitor: FBC.

Interactions: can ↑fx of oral hypoglycaemics. ↑risk of agranulocytosis with clozapine and toxicity with pentostatin.

Dose: specialist use only. NB: ↓dose if LF or RF.

☠ Stop immediately if rash or blood disorder occurs ☠.

CYCLOSPORIN see Ciclosporin

CYPROTERONE ACETATE

Anti-androgen; blocks androgen receptors. Also ↑s progestogens.
Use: Ca prostate[1] (as adjunct), acne[2] (esp 2° to PCOS, where often used with ethinylestradiol as co-cyprindiol), rarely for hypersexuality/sexual deviation[3] (*males only!*).
CI: (*none apply if for Ca prostate*) advanced DM (if vascular disease), sickle cell, malignancy/wasting diseases, Hx of TE, age <18 years (can ⇒ ↓bone/testicular development), severe depression, **L/P/B.**
SE: fatigue, gynaecomastia, ↑or ↓Wt, hepatotoxicity, blood disorders, hypersensitivity, osteoporosis, ↓spermatogenesis (reversible), TE, depression, carbohydrate metabolism and hair Δs.
Monitor: FBC, LFTs, adrenocortical function.
Warn: driving and other skilled tasks may be impaired.
Dose: 200–300 mg po daily in divided doses[1], 50 mg bd po[3].

▼ DABIGATRAN (ETEXILATE)/PRADAXA

Oral anticoagulant; direct thrombin inhibitor. Rapid onset and doesn't require therapeutic monitoring (unlike warfarin).
Use: Px of VTE after total knee or hip replacement.
CI: active bleeding, impaired haemostasis, **L** (if severe) **P/B.**
Caution: bleeding disorders, active GI ulceration, recent surgery, bacterial endocarditis, anaesthesia with postoperative indwelling epidural catheter (risk of paralysis; give initial dose ≥2 h after catheter removal and monitor for neurological signs), weight <50 kg, **R** (avoid if creatinine clearance <30 ml/min) **H/E.**
SE: haemorrhage, hepatobiliary disorders.
Monitor: for ↓Hb or signs of bleeding (stop drug if severe).
Interactions: NSAIDs ↑risk of bleeding. Levels ↑by amiodarone*.
Dose: 110 mg (75 mg if >75 years old) 1–4 h after surgery then 220 mg od (150 mg if >75 years old) for 9 days after knee replacement or 27–34 days after hip replacement. **NB: ↓dose in RF, elderly or if taking amiodarone*.**

▼ DALTEPARIN/FRAGMIN

Low-molecular-weight heparin (LMWH).

Use: DVT/PE Rx[1] and Px[2] (inc pre-operative), ACS (with aspirin)[3].

CI/Caution/SE/Monitor/Interactions: see Heparin.

Dose: *all sc*: 200 units/kg (max 18000 units) od[1]; 2500–5000 units od[2] (according to risk[SPC/BNF]) for ≥5 days; 120 units/kg bd[3] for ≥5 days (max 10000 units bd) reviewing dose if >8 days needed[SPC/BNF].

Consider monitoring anti Xa (3–4 h post dose) ± ↓dose if RF (i.e. creatinine >150), pregnancy, Wt >100 kg or <45 kg; see p. 212.

DANTRON

Stimulant laxative; theoretical risk of **carcinogenicity***.

Use: constipation (often limited to the terminally ill*).

Caution/SE: see Senna; possible carcinogenic risk. (CI if GI obstruction, **P/B**)

Dose: see Co-danthramer and Co-danthrusate.

DARBEPOETIN see Erythropoietin (recombinant form for ↓Hb).

DERMOVATE see Clobetasol propionate (steroid) cream 0.05%.

DESFERRIOXAMINE

Chelating agent; binds Fe (and Al) in gut ↓ing absorption/↑ing clearance.

Use: ↑Fe: acute (OD/poisoning[1]), chronic (e.g. xs transfusions for blood disorders, haemochromatosis when venesection CI). Also for ↑Al (e.g. 2° to dialysis).

Caution: Al-induced encephalopathy (may worsen), ↑risk of *Yersinia*/mucormycosis infection **R/P/B**.

SE: ↓BP (related to rate of ivi), lens opacities, retinopathy, GI upset, blood disorders, hypersensitivity. Also neurological/respiratory/renal dysfunction. ↑doses can ⇒ ↓growth and bone Δs.

Monitor: vision and hearing during chronic Rx.

Dose: acutely up to 15 mg/kg/h ivi (max 80 mg/kg/day)[1]. Otherwise according to degree of Fe or Al overload[SPC/BNF].

DEXAMETHASONE 0.1% EYE DROPS/MAXIDEX

Topical corticosteroid.

Use: uveitis, Px of post-eye surgery anterior segment inflammation.

CI: ocular infection.

SE: ocular infection (aggravation of existing or ↑susceptibility) or ocular HTN. If prolonged use, glaucoma and cataract possible.

Dose: 1 drop qds (max 1-hrly); specialist use only.

DEXAMETHASONE PHOSPHATE

Glucocorticoid; minimal mineralocorticoid activity, long duration of action (see p. 225).

Use: cerebral oedema (from malignancy), spinal cord compression, Dx of Cushing's, N&V (2° to chemotherapy or surgery), allergy/inflammation (esp if unresponsive shock), congenital adrenal hyperplasia, rheumatic disease.

CI/Caution/SE/Warn/Interactions: see Prednisolone and steroids section (p. 225).

Dose: cerebral oedema: acutely 10 mg iv, then 4 mg im qds 2–4 days (if not life-threatening, some go straight to 4 mg qds iv then switch to po a few days later, stopped gradually over 5–7 days). For other indications, see SPC/BNF.

☠Doses given here are for dexamethasone phosphate and must be prescribed as such: other forms have different doses☠!

DF118 (suffix FORTE often omitted) Dihydrocodeine 40 mg.

Dose: 40–80 mg tds po.

NB: tablets are different dose to non-proprietary dihydrocodeine.

DIAMORPHINE (HEROIN HYDROCHLORIDE)

Strong opiate (1.5 × strength of morphine if both given iv).

Use: severe pain (acute and chronic)[1], AMI[2], acute LVF[3].

CI/Caution/SE/Interactions: as morphine, but less nausea/↓BP, and does not interact with baclofen, gabapentin and ritonavir.

☠ **Respiratory depression** (esp elderly) ☠

Dose: 5–10 mg sc/im (or 1/4–1/2 this dose iv) up to 4-hrly[1]; 5 mg iv (at 1–2 mg/min) followed by further 2.5–5 mg if necessary[2], 2.5–5 mg iv (at 1 mg/min)[3]. Can give via sc pump in chronic pain/palliative care: see p. 189. **NB:** ↓dose if elderly, LF or RF.

DIAZEMULS iv diazepam emulsion: ⇒ ↓venous irritation.

DIAZEPAM

Benzodiazepine, long-acting.
Use: seizures (esp status epilepticus[1], febrile convulsions), *short-term* Rx of acute alcohol withdrawal[2], anxiety[3], insomnia[4] (if also anxiety; if not, then shorter-acting forms preferred as ⇒ ↓hangover sedation). Also used for muscle spasm[5].
CI: respiratory depression, marked neuromuscular respiratory weakness inc unstable myasthenia gravis, sleep apnoea, acute pulmonary insufficiency, chronic psychosis, depression (don't give diazepam alone), **L** (if severe).
Caution: respiratory disease, muscle weakness (inc MG), Hx of drug/alcohol abuse, personality disorder, porphyria, R/P/B/E.
SE: respiratory depression (rarely apnoea), drowsiness, dependence. Also ataxia, amnesia, headache, vertigo, GI upset, jaundice, ↓BP, ↓HR, visual/libido/urinary disturbances, blood disorders, paradoxical disinhibition in Ψ disorder.
Warn: sedation ↑by alcohol and ⇒ ↓driving/skilled task ability.
Interactions: metab by **P450** ∴ many: ery-/clari-/-teli-thromycin, quinu-/dalfo-pristin and flu-/itra-/keto-/posa-conazole can ↑levels. Sedative fx ↑by antipsychotics, antidepressants, antiepileptics and antiretrovirals. Can ↑fx of zidovudine and sodium oxybate. ↑risk of ↓HR/BP and respiratory depression with im olanzapine.
Dose: for status epilepticus[1] and alcohol withdrawal[2], see p. 252 and p. 195, respectively; 2 mg tds po (↑up to 30 mg/day)[3,5]; 5–15 mg nocte po[4]. **NB:** ↓dose if elderly, LF or RF. If chronic exposure to benzodiazepines, ↑doses may be needed; don't stop suddenly, as can ⇒ withdrawal; see p. 229 for details.

> 💀 **Respiratory depression:** if ↑doses used (esp iv/im), monitor O_2 sats and have O_2 ($\pm$ intubation equipment) at hand, caution with flumazenil – see p. 256 for Mx 💀.

DICLOFENAC

Medium-strength NSAID; non-selective COX inhibitor.

Use: pain/inflammation, esp musculoskeletal; RA, osteoarthritis, acute gout, migraine, post-op and dental pain.

CI/Caution/SE/Interactions: as ibuprofen, but somewhat ↑risk PU/GI bleeds & thrombotic events (↓risk PU/GI bleeds if given with misoprostol as Arthrotec). Doses $\geq$ 150 mg daily associated with ↑thrombotic risk. Avoid in acute porphyria. Ciclosporin ⇒ ↑serum levels. No known interaction with baclofen. Mild **W** +.

Dose: 25–50 mg tds po or 75 mg bd po (or im, but for max of 2 days); 75–150 mg/day pr (**divided doses**). Rarely used iv[BNF/SPC]. MR and top preparations available[BNF/SPC]. **NB: Avoid/ ↓dose in RF & consider gastroprotective Rx.**

DIFFLAM Benzydamine: topical NSAID for painful inflammatory conditions of oropharynx (e.g. mouth ulcers, radio-/chemo-therapy-induced mucositis). Available as spray (4–8 sprays 1.5–3-hrly) or oral rinse (15 ml 1.5–3-hrly, diluting in 15 ml water if stinging). Rarely ⇒ hypersensitivity reactions.

DIGIBIND Anti-digoxin Ab for digoxin toxicity/OD unresponsive to supportive Rx. See SPC for dose.

DIGOXIN

Cardiac glycoside: ↓s HR by slowing AVN conduction and ↑ing vagal tone. Also weak inotrope.

Use: AF (and other SVTs), HF.

CI: HB (intermittent complete), 2nd-degree AV block, VF, VT, HOCM (can use with care if also AF and HF), SVTs 2° to WPW.

Caution: recent MI, ↓K⁺*/↓T₄ (both ⇒ ↑digoxin sensitivity*), SSS, rhythms resembling AF (e.g. atrial tachycardia with variable AV block), **R/E** (↓dose), **P**.

SE: generally mild unless rapid ivi, xs Rx or OD: **GI upset** (esp nausea), **arrhythmias/HB, neuro-Ψ disturbances** (inc visual Δs, esp blurred vision and yellow/green halos), fatigue, weakness, confusion, hallucinations, mood Δs. Also gynaecomastia (if chronic Rx), rarely ↓Pt, rash, ↑EØ.

Monitor: U&Es, digoxin levels (ideally take 6 h post-Dose: therapeutic range = 1–2 microgram/l).

Interactions: digoxin fx/toxicity ↑d by Ca²⁺ antagonists (esp verapamil), amiodarone, propafenone, quinidine, antimalarials, itraconazole, amphotericin, ciclosporin, St John's wort and diuretics (mostly via ↓K⁺*), but also ACE-i/ARBs and spironolactone (despite potential ↑K⁺). Cholestyramine and antacids can ↓digoxin absorption.

Dose: *non-acute AF/SVTs:* load with 125–250 microgram bd po (maintenance dose 62.5–250 microgram od). For HF: 62.5–125 microgram od. **NB: ↓dose if RF, elderly or digoxin given <2 wks ago.**

Digoxin loading for acute AF/SVTs: *either* 0.75–1 mg as ivi over 2 h *or* 500 microgram po repeated 12 h later. Then follow non-acute schedule.

DIHYDROCODEINE see Codeine: similar-strength opioid.

Dose: 30 mg 4–6 hourly po (or up to 50 mg 4–6 hourly im/sc) with or after food. ↑doses can be given under close supervision. ↓dose if RF.

DILATING EYE DROPS (for funduscopy). Generally safe but rarely ⇒ angle closure glaucoma (suspect if develops red painful eye with ↓vision and nausea; *ophthalmic emergency*). Dilation blurs vision. Driving unsafe for at least 4 hours when both eyes dilated. Apply 1 drop and allow 15 mins for effect.

1 **Tropicamide 1%** Most common; CI in children <1 yr old (use 0.5%).
2 **Phenylephrine 2.5% or 10%** Frequently used in combination with tropicamide. 2.5% most common. 10% ↑s systemic SEs. CI if cardiac disease, HTN, ↑HR, aneurysms, ↑T₄.

Consider cycloplegic forms (e.g. cyclopentolate 1%) for refraction in children or if analgesia required, e.g. corneal abrasions & uveitis (↓s ciliary spasm).

DILTIAZEM

Rate-limiting benzothiazepine Ca^{2+} channel blocker: ↓s HR and contractility* (but < verapamil) and ↓s BP. Also dilates peripheral/coronary arteries.

Use: Rx/Px of angina[1] (esp if β-blockers CI) and HTN[2] *(for advice on stepped HTN Mx see p. 182)*.

CI: LVF* with pulmonary congestion, ↓↓HR, 2nd/3rd-degree AV block (without pacemaker), SSS, acute porphyria **P/B**.

Caution: 1st-degree AV block, ↓HR, ↑PR interval, **L/R/H**.

SE: headache, flushing, GI upset (esp N&C), oedema (esp ankle), ↓HR, ↓BP, gum hyperplasia. Rarely SAN/AVN block, arrhythmias, rash, hepatotoxicity, gynaecomastia.

Interactions: β-blockers and verapamil (can ⇒ asystole, AV block, ↓↓HR, HF). ↑s fx of digoxin, ciclosporin, theophyllines, carbamazepine and phenytoin. ☠ ↑risk of VF with iv dandrolene ☠.

Dose: 60 mg tds (↑ing to max of 360 mg/day)[1]; 180–480 mg/day in 1 or 2 doses[2] (suitable for HTN only as MR preparation: no non-proprietary forms exist and brands vary in clinical fx ∴ specify which is required[SPC/BNF]). **NB: Consider ↓ing doses if LF or RF.**

DIPROBASE Paraffin-based emollient cream/ointment for dry skin conditions (e.g. eczema, psoriasis).

DIPYRIDAMOLE/PERSANTIN

Antiplatelet agent: inhibits Pt aggregation, adhesion and survival (also ⇒ arterial dilation: inc coronaries).

Use: 2° prevention of ischaemic TIA/CVA[1], Px of TE from prosthetic valves (as adjunct to warfarin)[2].

Caution: recent MI, angina (if unstable), aortic stenosis, coagulation disorders, ↓BP, MG*, migraine (may worsen), **H/B**.

SE: GI upset, dizziness, myalgia, headache, ↓BP, ↑HR, hot flushes, rarely worsening of IHD, hypersensitivity (rash, urticaria, bronchospasm, angioedema), ↑postoperative bleeding, ↓Pt.

Interactions: ↓s fx (but ↑s hypotensive fx) of cholinesterase inhibitors*, ↑s fx of adenosine. **W +** .

Dose: 200 mg bd po as MR preparation (**Persantin retard**)[1,2]; 100–200 mg tds po[2]. All doses to be taken with food.

DISODIUM ETIDRONATE see Pamidronate.

DISODIUM PAMIDRONATE see Pamidronate.

DISULFIRAM/ANTABUSE

Alcohol dehydrogenase inhibitor: $\Rightarrow$ ↑systemic acetaldehyde $\Rightarrow$ unpleasant SE when alcohol ingested (inc small amounts ∴ care with alcohol-containing medications, foods, toiletries).
Use: alcohol withdrawal (maintenance of).
CI: Hx of IHD or CVA, HTN, psychosis, ↑suicide risk, severe personality disorder, **H/P/B**.
Caution: DM, epilepsy, respiratory disease, **L/R**.
SE: only if alcohol ingested – N&V, flushing, headache, ↑HR, ↓BP ($\pm$ collapse if xs alcohol intake).
Interactions: ↑s fx of phenytoin, ↑toxicity with paraldehyde **W +**.
Dose: initially 800 mg od, ↓ing to 100–200 mg od over 5 days. Review if >6 months.

NB: Must have consumed no alcohol within at least 24 h of 1st dose. Prescribe under specialist supervision.

DOBUTAMINE

Inotropic sympathomimetic: mostly β_1 fx $\Rightarrow$ ↑contractility. ↓fx on HR compared with dopamine.
Use: shock (cardiogenic, septic).
Caution: severe ↓BP.
SE: ↑HR, ↑BP (if xs Rx), phlebitis, ↓Pt.
Interactions: risk of ↑BP crisis with β-blockers (esp if 'non-selective').
Dose: 2.5–10 microgram/kg/min ivi, titrating to response (via central line, preferably with invasive cardiac monitoring). Often given with dopamine; seek expert help.

DOCUSATE SODIUM

Stimulant laxative: ⇒ ↑GI motility (also a softening agent).
Use/Caution/SE: see Senna (**CI if GI obstruction**).
Dose: 50–100 mg up to tds po (max 500 mg/day). Also available as enemas[SPC/BNF].

DOMPERIDONE

Antiemetic: D_2 antagonist – inhibits central nausea chemoreceptor trigger zone. Poor BBB penetration ∴ ↓central SEs (extrapyramidal fx, sedation) cf other dopamine antagonists.
Use: N&V, esp 2° to chemotherapy or 'morning-after pill', and in Parkinson's disease or migraine. Rarely for gastro-oesophageal reflux and dyspepsia.
CI: prolactinoma, when GI obstruction harmful, **L**.
Caution: GI obstruction **R/P/B**.
SE: rash, allergy, ↑prolactin (can ⇒ gynaecomastia, galactorrhoea and hyperprolactinoma). Rarely ↓libido, dystonia and extrapyramidal fx.
Dose: 10 mg tds po (can ↑to max 20 mg qds); 60 mg bd pr. Not available im/iv. **NB:** ↓dose if RF.

DONEPEZIL/ARICEPT

Acetylcholinesterase inhibitor (reversible); see Rivastigmine.
Use: Alzheimer's disease: mild or moderate[NICE].
CI: **P/B**.
Caution: supraventricular conduction dfx (esp SSS), ↑risk of PU (e.g. Hx of PU or NSAID), COPD/asthma, extrapyramidal symptoms can worsen, **L**.
SE: **cholinergic fx** (see p. 233), **GI upset** (esp initially), **insomnia** (if occurs, change dose to mane), **headache**, fatigue, dizziness, syncope, rash, Ψ disturbances. Rarely ↓ or ↑BP, seizures, PU/GI bleeds, SAN/AVN block, hepatotoxicity.
Interactions: metab by **P450** ∴ inhibitors and inducers on p. 237 could ↑ or ↓ levels, respectively; check BNF/SPC.

Dose: 5 mg nocte (↑to 10 mg after 1 month if necessary); specialist use only – need review for clinical response and tolerance. Continue only if MMSE remains 10–20[NICE].

DOPAMINE

Inotropic sympathomimetic: dose-dependent fx on receptors: low doses (2–3 microgram/kg/min) stimulate peripheral DA receptors but little else ∴ ⇒ ↑renal perfusion*; higher doses (>5 microgram/kg/min) also have β_1 fx (⇒ ↑contractility); even higher doses have α fx (⇒ vasoconstriction, but can worsen HF).

Use: shock, esp if AKI* or cardiogenic (e.g. post-MI or cardiac surgery).

CI: tachyarrhythmias, phaeo, ↑T_4.

Caution: correct hypovolaemia before giving.

SE: N&V, ↓ or ↑BP, ↑HR, peripheral vasoconstriction.

Interactions: fx ↑by cyclopropane and halogen hydrocarbon anaesthetics (are CI) or MAOIs (can ⇒ ↑↑BP; consider ↓↓dose of dopamine).

Dose: initially 2–5 microgram/kg/min ivi (via central line, preferably with invasive cardiac monitoring), then adjust to response; seek specialist help.

DORZOLAMIDE/TRUSOPT

Topical carbonic anhydrase inhibitor: as acetazolamide (oral preparation, which is more potent but has ↑SEs*).

Use: glaucoma (esp if β-blocker or PG analogue CI or fails to ↓IOP).

CI: ↑Cl^- acidosis, **R** (severe only), **P/B**.

Caution: Hx of renal stones[†], **L**.

SE: local irritation & allergic reactions, blurred vision, bitter taste, rash. Rarely* systemic SEs (esp urolithiasis[†]) and interactions; see Acetazolamide.

Dose: apply 2% drop bd/tds. Available as combination drop with timolol 0.5% (Cosopt).

DOXAPRAM

Respiratory stimulant: $\uparrow$s activity of respiratory and vasomotor centres in medulla $\Rightarrow$ $\uparrow$depth (and, to lesser extent, rate) of breathing. Also indirect fx by stimulation of chemoreceptors in aorta and carotid artery.

Use: hypoventilation, life-threatening respiratory failure – usually only if dt transient/reversible cause, e.g. post-operative/-general anaesthetic or acute deterioration with known precipitant. Mostly used in preventing respiratory depression $2°$ to $\uparrow FiO_2$ used in severe respiratory acidosis (can be harmful if CO_2 $\downarrow$ or normal).

CI: severe asthma or HTN, IHD, $\uparrow T_4$, epilepsy, physical obstruction of respiratory tract.

Caution: if taking MAOIs, **L/H/P**.

SE: headache, flushing, chest pains, arrhythmias, vasoconstriction, $\uparrow$BP, $\uparrow$HR, laryngo-/broncho-spasm, cough, salivation, GI upset, dizziness, seizures.

Dose: specialist use only (mostly in ITU).

DOXAZOSIN/CARDURA

α_1-Blocker $\Rightarrow$ systemic vasodilation and relaxation of internal urethral sphincter $\therefore$ $\Rightarrow$ $\downarrow$TPR[1] and $\uparrow$bladder outflow[2].

Use: HTN[1] (*for advice on stepped HTN Mx see p. 182*), BPH[2].

CI: **B**.

Caution: postural $\downarrow$BP, micturition syncope, **L/H/P/E**.

SE: postural $\downarrow$BP (esp after 1st dose*), **dizziness, headache, urinary incontinence** (esp women), GI upset (esp N&V), drowsiness/fatigue, syncope, mood Δs, dry mouth, oedema, somnolence, blurred vision, rhinitis. Rarely erectile dysfunction, $\uparrow$HR, arrhythmias, hypersensitivity/rash. Chronic Rx $\Rightarrow$ beneficial lipid Δs ($\uparrow$HDL, $\downarrow$LDL, $\downarrow$VLDL, $\downarrow$TG, $\downarrow$Pt, $\downarrow$NØ).

Interactions: $\uparrow$s hypotensive fx of diuretics, β-blockers, Ca^{2+} antagonists, silden-/tadal-/varden-afil, general anaesthetics, moxisylyte and antidepressants.

Dose: initially 1 mg od (give 1st dose before bed*), then slowly $\uparrow$according to response (max 16 mg/day[1] or 8 mg/day[2]). 4 mg or 8 mg od if MR preparation, as Cardura XL.

DOXYCYCLINE

Tetracycline antibiotic: inhibits ribosomal (30S) subunit. Has longest $t_{1/2}$ of all tetracyclines $\therefore$ od dosing.

Use: genital infections, esp syphilis, chlamydia, PID, salpingitis, urethritis (non-gonococcal). Also *Rickettsia* (inc Q fever), *Brucella*, Lyme disease (*Borrelia burgdorferi*), malaria (Px/Rx, not 1st-line), mycoplasma (genital/respiratory), COPD infective exac (*H. influenzae*), **MRSA** infection (if mild, sensitive strain).

CI/Caution/SE/Interactions: as tetracycline, but can give with caution if RF, although is also CI in SLE and achlorhydria. Can $\Rightarrow$ anorexia, flushing, tinnitus and can ↑ciclosporin levels.

Warn: avoid UV light and Zn-/Fe-containing products (e.g. antacids).

Dose: 100–200 mg od/bd[SPC/BNF]. **NB:** ↓dose in RF.

▼ DULOXETINE/CYMBALTA[1,2,3] OR YENTREVE[4]

5HT and noradrenaline reuptake inhibitor.

Use: depression[1] (see p. 197), generalised anxiety disorder[2], diabetic neuropathy[3] (review need ≤3 monthly and stop if inadequate response after 2 months), stress urinary incontinence[4] (assess benefit/tolerability after 2–4 wks).

CI: R (avoid if creatinine clearance <30 ml/min) **L/P/B**.

Caution: cardiac disease, Hx of mania or seizures, ↑IOP, susceptibility to angle closure glaucoma, bleeding disorders/on drugs ↑ing bleeding risk, **H/P/B/E**.

SE: N&V&C, abdominal pain, dyspepsia, WtΔ, ↓appetite, palpitations, hot flushes, insomnia, sexual dysfunction, suicidal behaviour.

Interactions: metabolism ↓by ciprofloxacin, fluvoxamine. ↑5HT fx with St John's wort and antidepressants (esp moclobemide and MAOIs; avoid concomitant use and don't start for 1 wk after stopping duloxetine). Avoid with artemether/lumefantrine. ↑risk CNS toxicity with sibutramine.

Warn: patient not to stop suddenly*

Dose: 60 mg od[1]; initially 30 mg od (↑to max 120 mg/day if required)[2]; 60 mg od (↑to bd if required)[3]; 40 mg bd[4].

NB: stop gradually over 1–2 wks to ↓risk of withdrawal fx* (see p. 235).

EDROPHONIUM

Short-acting cholinesterase antagonist, given iv during Tensilon test for Dx of MG: look for ↓signs (e.g. ↑power, ↓ptosis).

ENALAPRIL/INNOVACE

ACE-i.
Use: HTN[1] (*for advice on stepped HTN Mx see p. 182*), LVF[2].
CI/Caution/SE/Interactions: as Captopril, plus **L**.
Dose: initially 5 mg od[1] (2.5 mg od[2]) ↑ing according to response max 40 mg/day. NB: ↓dose elderly, taking diuretics or RF.

ENOXAPARIN/CLEXANE

Low-molecular-weight heparin (LMWH).
Use: DVT/PE Rx[1] and Px[2] (inc pre-operative), ACS (with aspirin)[3].
CI/Caution/SE/Monitor/Interactions: as Heparin, plus **B**.
Dose: (all sc; 1 mg = 100 units) 1.5 mg/kg od[1], 40 mg od (20 mg od if not high risk)[2], 1 mg/kg bd[3].

Consider monitoring anti-Xa (3–4 h post dose) and ↓dose if RF (i.e. creatinine >150), pregnancy, Wt >100 kg or <45 kg; see p. 212.

ENSURE Protein and calorie supplement drinks.

EPADERM Paraffin-based emollient ointment for very dry skin (and as soap substitute).

EPILIM see Valproate.

EPINEPHRINE see Adrenaline.

EPOETIN see Erythropoietin (recombinant form for ↓Hb).

EPROSARTAN/TEVETEN

Angiotensin II antagonist; see Losartan.
L ∴: HTN (*for advice on stepped HTN Mx see p. 182*)
CI: L (if severe), **P/B**.
Caution/SE/Interactions: see Losartan.

Dose: 600 mg od (max 800 mg od). Start at 300 mg and then ↑as required if elderly, RF or LF.

EPTIFIBATIDE/INTEGRILIN

Antiplatelet agent: glycoprotein IIb/IIIa receptor inhibitor – stops binding of fibrinogen and inhibits platelet aggregation.
Use: Px of MI in unstable angina or NSTEMI (if last episode of chest pain w/in 24 h), esp if high risk and awaiting PCI[NICE] (see p. 240).
CI: haemorrhagic diathesis, severe trauma or major surgery w/in 6 wks, abnormal bleeding or CVA w/in 30 days, Hx of haemorrhagic CVA or intracranial disease (AVM, aneurysm or neoplasm), ↓Pt, ↑INR, severe HTN, **L** (if significant), **R** (if severe), **B**.
Caution: drugs that ↑bleeding risk (esp thrombolysis), **P**.
SE: bleeding.
Monitor: FBC (baseline, w/in 6 h of giving, then at least daily) plus clotting and creatinine (baseline at least).
Dose: initially 180 microgram/kg iv bolus followed by ivi of 2 microgram/kg/min for up to 72 h (or 96 h if PCI during treatment). NB: needs concurrent heparin and ↓dose if RF[SPC/BNF].

Specialist use only: get senior advice or contact on-call cardiology.

ERGOCALCIFEROL (= CALCIFEROL)

Vit D_2: needs renal (1) and hepatic (25) hydroxylation for activation.
Use: vitamin D deficiency.
CI: ↑Ca^{2+}, metastatic calcification.
Caution: **R** (if high 'pharmacological'* doses used), **B**.
SE: ↑Ca^{2+}. If over-Rx: **GI upset**, weakness, headache, polydipsia/polyuria, anorexia, RF, arrhythmias.
Monitor: Ca^{2+} (esp if N&V develops or ↑doses in RF*).
Interactions: fx ↓by anticonvulsants and ↑by thiazides.
Dose: 10–20 microgram (400–800 units) od as part of multivitamin preparations or combined with calcium lactate or phosphate as 'calcium + ergocalciferol': non-proprietary preparations available but is often prescribed by trade name (e.g. Cacit D3, or Calcichew D3). ↑doses of 0.25–1.0 mg od (of 'pharmacological strength'

preparations*) used for GI malabsorption and chronic liver disease
(up to 5 mg daily for ↓PTH or renal osteodystrophy).

*Specify strength of tablet required to avoid confusion[SPC/BNF].

ERYTHROMYCIN

Macrolide antibiotic: binds 50S ribosome.

Use: atypical pneumonias (with other agents; see p. 172), rarely
Chlamydia/other GU infections, *Campylobacter* enteritis. Often used if
allergy to penicillin.

CI: macrolide hypersensitivity or if taking terfenadine, pimozide,
ergotamine or dihydroergotamine.

Caution: ↑QTc (inc drugs that predispose to), porphyria, **L/R/P/B**.

SE: GI upset (rarely AAC), **dry itchy skin**, hypersensitivity (inc SJS,
TEN), arrhythmias (esp VT), chest pain, reversible hearing loss (dose-
related, esp if RF), cholestatic jaundice.

Interactions: ↓P450 ∴ many; most importantly ↑s levels of
ciclosporin, digoxin, theophyllines and carbamazepine, **W** + .

Dose: 500 mg qds po (250 mg qds if mild infection, 1 g qds if severe);
50 mg/kg daily iv in 4 divided doses.

NB: venous irritant ∴ give po if possible.

ERYTHROPOIETIN

Recombinant erythropoietin.

Use: ↓Hb 2° to CRF or chemotherapy (AZT or platinum-containing).
Also unlicensed use for myeloma, lymphoma and certain myelodys-
plasias. 3 types: α (Eprex), β (NeoRecormon) and longer-acting
darbepoetin (Aranesp).

SE: ↑BP, ↑K+, headache, arthralgia, oedema, TE. ☠Rarely ⇒ red
cell aplasia (esp subcutaneous Eprex if RF, which is now CI)☠.

CI/Caution/Dose: specialist use only[SPC/BNF]; given subcutaneously
(self-administered) or iv (as inpatient). ↓Fe/folate (monitor), ↑Al,
infections and inflammatory disease can ↓response. NB: *transfusion is
1st-line Rx for ↓Hb 2° to cancer chemotherapy.*

ESCITALOPRAM/CIPRALEX

SSRI (active enantiomer of citalopram).
Use: Depression (see p. 197), OCD, anxiety disorders.
CI/Caution/SE/Warn/Interactions: as citalopram.
Dose: initially 10 mg od, ↑ing if necessary to 20 mg od. **NB: max dose 10 mg in elderly and halve doses in LF and for most anxiety disorders.**

ESMOLOL

β-blocker: cardioselective ($\beta_1 > \beta_2$) and short-acting*.
Use: SVTs (inc AF, atrial flutter, sinus ↑HR), HTN (esp peri-operatively), acute MI (*safer than long-acting preparations).
CI/Caution/SE/Interactions: see Propranolol.
Dose: usually 50–200 microgram/kg/min ivi, preceded by loading dose if perioperative[SPC].

ESOMEPRAZOLE/NEXIUM

PPI; as Omeprazole, plus **R** (if severe).
Dose: 20 mg od po (40 mg od for 1st 4 wks, if for gastro-oesophageal reflux); 20–40 mg/day iv[SPC/BNF](▼).
NB: Max 20 mg/day if severe LF.

ETANERCEPT/ENBREL

Monoclonal Ab against TNF-α (an inflammatory cytokine).
Use: severe arthritis (rheumatoid[NICE], juvenile idiopathic[NICE] and psoriatic), severe plaque psoriasis[NICE] and ankylosing spondylitis[NICE].
CI/Caution/Interactions: See SPC.
SE: blood disorders, severe infections, CNS demyelination, GI upset, exac of HF, headache. *Specialist use only.*

☠ Don't give live vaccines during Rx. Risk of infections (e.g. TB, inc extrapulmonary) and theoretical malignancy risk ☠.

ETHAMBUTOL

Anti-TB antibiotic: inhibits cell-wall synthesis ('static').
Use: TB initial Rx phase (1st 2 months) *if isoniazid resistance known or suspected* (see pp. 175).

CI: optic neuritis, ↓vision.
Caution: **R** (monitor levels* and ↓dose if creatinine clearance <30 ml/min), **P/E**.
SE: neuritis; peripheral and **optic** (can ⇒ ↓visual acuity**, colour-blindness, ↓visual fields ∴ ⇒ baseline and regular ophthalmology review). Rarely GI upset, skin reactions, ↓Pt.
Warn: patient to report immediately any visual symptoms – use alternative drug if unable to do this (e.g. very young, ↓IQ).
Monitor: visual acuity** (inc baseline before Rx), plasma levels*.
Dose: 15 mg/kg od (30 mg/kg 3 times a week if 'supervised' Rx)[SPC/BNF].
NB: ↓dose if RF.

▼ ETORICOXIB/ARCOXIA

NSAID which selectively inhibits COX-2 ∴ ↓GI SEs (COX-1 mediated). *Provides no Px against IHD/CVA (unlike aspirin).*
Use: osteo[1]/rheumatoid[2] arthritis[NICE], ankylosing spondylitis[2], acute gout[3].
CI/Caution/SE/Interactions: as celecoxib (except fluconazole interaction), plus CI in uncontrolled HTN (persistently >140/90 mmHg) – monitor BP w/in 2 wks of starting & regularly thereafter. Also ↑s ethinylestradiol levels. *Not* CI in *sulphonamide* hyper-sensitivity. Mild [**W** +].
Dose: 30–60 mg od[1]; 90 mg od[2]; 120 mg od[3] for max 8 days. **NB:** ↓dose if LF.

EUMOVATE see Clobetasone butyrate 0.05%; steroid cream.

FANSIDAR

Antimalarial: combination tablet of pyrimethamine (25 mg) + sulfadoxine (500 mg).
Use: Rx of falciparum malaria (with or following quinine).
CI: sulphonamide or pyrimethamine allergy, porphyria.
Caution: blood disorders, asthma, G6PD deficiency, **L/R/P/B/E**.
SE: blood disorders, skin reactions*, pulmonary infiltrates, insomnia, GI upset, nephrotoxicity, hepatotoxicity, hypersensitivity.

Monitor: FBC (if chronic Rx) and for rash* or cough/SOB (stop drug).
Dose: see BNF/SPC.

FELODIPINE/PLENDIL

Ca^{2+} channel blocker (dihydropyridine): as amlodipine but $\Rightarrow$ ↓HF/–ve inotropic fx.
Use: HTN[1] (*for advice on stepped Mx see p. 182*), angina Px[2].
CI: IHD (if unstable angina or w/in 1 month of MI), significant aortic stenosis, acute porphyria, **H** (if uncontrolled)/**P**.
Caution: stop drug if angina/HF worsen, **L/B**.
SE: as nifedipine but ↑ankle swelling and possibly ↓vasodilator fx (headache, flushing and dizziness).
Interactions: metab by **P450** ∴ levels ↑by cimetidine, erythromycin, ketoconazole and **grapefruit juice**. Hypotensive fx ↑by α-blockers. Levels ↓by primidone. ↑s fx of tacrolimus.
Dose: initially 5 mg od, ↑if required to 10 mg (max 20 mg[1]).
NB: ↓dose if LF or elderly.

FENTANYL

Strong opioid; used in severe chronic/palliative pain (top/sl/buccal/nasal spray) and in anaesthesia (iv).
CI: acute respiratory depression, risk of ileus, ↑ICP/head injury/coma.
Caution: all other conditions where morphine is CI or cautioned, but better tolerated in RF. Also DM, cerebral tumour.
SE: as morphine but generally ↓N&V/constipation.
Interactions: as morphine but levels ↑(not ↓) by ritonavir, levels ↑by itra-/flu-conazole & no known interaction with gabapentin. May ↑levels of midazolam.
Warn: patients/carers of signs/symptoms of opiate toxicity.
Dose: Patches: last 72 h and come in 5 strengths: 12, 25, 50, 75 and 100, which denote release of microgram/h (to calculate initial dose, these are approx equivalent to daily oral morphine requirement of 45, 90, 180, 270 and 360 mg, respectively).

Lozenges (buccal) for 'breakthrough' pain as Actiq: initially 200 microgram over 15 min, repeating after 15 min if needed and adjusting dose to give max 4 lozenges daily (available as 200, 400, 600, 800, 1200 or 1600 microgram).

Tablets: for 'breakthrough' pain as ▼ Effentora (buccal) or ▼ Abstral(sl) 100, 200, 400, 600 and 800 microgram[SPC/BNF]. *Only use if taking regular opioids (fatalities reported otherwise). If >4 doses/day needed, adjust background analgesia.*

Nasal spray: for 'breakthrough' pain as ▼ Instanyl or ▼ PecFent[SPC/BNF]. **NB: ↓dose if LF or elderly. No initial ↓dose needed in RF, but may accumulate over time. Unless given iv has prolonged onset/offset; use only when opioid requirements stable & cover 1st 12 hrs after initial Rx with prn short acting opioid.** Only for use if have previously tolerated opioids. If serious adverse reactions remove patch immediately and monitor for up to 24 h. Fever/external heat can ⇒ ↑absorption (∴ ↑fx) from patches.

FERROUS FUMARATE

As ferrous sulphate, but ↓GI upset; available in UK as Fersaday (322-mg tablet od as Px or bd as Rx), Fersamal (1–2 tablets of 210 mg tds) or Galfer (305 mg capsule od/bd).

FERROUS GLUCONATE

As ferrous sulphate, but ↓GI upset. Px: 600 mg od; Rx: 1.2–1.8 g/day in 2–3 divided doses.

FERROUS SULPHATE

Oral Fe preparation.
Use: Fe-deficient ↓Hb Rx/Px.
Caution: P.
SE: dark stools (can confuse with melaena, which smells worse!), GI upset (esp nausea; consider switching to ferrous gluconate/fumarate or take with food, but latter can ⇒ ↓absorption), Δ bowel habit (dose-dependent).
Dose: Rx: 200 mg bd/tds. Px: 200 mg od.

FINASTERIDE

Antiandrogen: 5-α-reductase inhibitor; ↓s testosterone conversion to more potent dihydrotestosterone.
Use: BPH[1] (↓s prostate size and symptoms), male-pattern baldness[2].
Caution: Ca prostate (can ⇒ ↓PSA and ∴ mask), obstructive uropathy, **P** (teratogenic; although not taken by women, partners of those on the drug can absorb it from handling crushed tablets and from semen, in which it is excreted ∴ *females must avoid handling tablets, and sexual partners of those on the drug must use condoms if, or likely to become, pregnant*).
SE: sexual dysfunction, testicular pain, gynaecomastia, hypersensitivity (inc swelling of lips/face).
Dose: 5 mg od[1] (Proscar), 1 mg od[2] (Propecia).

FLAGYL see Metronidazole; antibiotic for anaerobes

FLECAINIDE

Class Ic antiarrhythmic; local anaesthetic; ↓s conduction.
Use: VT[1] (if serious and symptomatic), SVT[2] (esp junctional re-entry tachycardias and paroxysmal AF).
CI: SAN dysfunction, atrial conduction dfx, HB (not 1st-degree), BBB, AF post-cardiac surgery, chronic AF (with no attempts at cardioversion), Hx of MI plus asymptomatic VEs or non-sustained VT, valvular heart disease (if haemodynamically compromised), **H**.
Caution: pacemakers, ensure e'lytes normalised before use, **L/R/P/B/E**.
SE: GI upset, syncope, dyspnoea, vision/mood disturbances. Rarely arrhythmias.
Monitor: pre-dose plasma levels in LF or RF (keep at 0.2–1 mg/l), ECG if giving iv.
Interactions: levels ↑d by amiodarone, ritonavir, fluoxetine and quinine. ↑s digoxin levels. Myocardial depression may occur with β-blockers/verapamil. ↑risk of arrhythmias with antipsychotics, TCAs, artemether/lumefantrine and dolasetron.
Dose: initially 100 mg bd po, ↓ing after 3–5 days if possible (max 400 mg/day)[1]; 50 mg bd po, ↑ing if necessary to 300 mg/day[2].

Acutely, 2 mg/kg iv over 10–30 min (max 150 mg), then (if required) 1.5 mg/kg/h ivi for 1 h, then ↓ing to 100–250 microgram/kg/h for up to 24 h, then give po (max cumulative dose in 1st 24 h = 600 mg). NB: ↓dose if LF/RF.

FLEET (PHOSPHO-SODA) see Bowel preparations.
Dose: 45 ml (mixed with 120 ml water, then followed by 240 ml water) taken twice: for morning procedures, at 7 am and 7 pm the day before; for afternoon procedures, at 7 pm the day before and at 7 am on the day of procedure.

FLIXOTIDE see Fluticasone (inh steroid). 50, 100, 250 or 500 microgram/puff as powder. 50, 125 or 250 microgram/puff as aerosol.
Dose: 100–2000 microgram/day[SPC/BNF] (aerosol doses ? < powder doses).

FLOMAXTRA XL see Tamsulosin; α_1-blocker for ↑prostate.

FLUCLOXACILLIN

Penicillin (penicillinase-resistant).
Use: penicillin-resistant (β-lactamase-producing) staphylococcal infections, esp skin[1] (surgical wounds, iv sites, cellulitis, impetigo, otitis externa), rarely as adjunct in pneumonia[1]. Also osteomyelitis[2], endocarditis[3].
CI/Caution/SE/Interactions: as benzylpenicillin, plus CI if Hx of flucloxacillin-associated jaundice/hepatic dysfunction and caution if LF, as rarely ⇒ hepatitis or **cholestatic jaundice** (may develop up to 2 months after Rx stopped).
Dose: 250–500 mg qds po/im (or up to 2 g qds iv)[1]; up to 2 g qds iv[2]; 2 g qds (4-hrly if Wt > 85 kg) iv[3].
NB: ↓dose in severe RF.

FLUCONAZOLE

Triazole antifungal: good po absorption and CSF penetration.
Use: fungal meningitis (esp cryptococcal), candidiasis (mucosal, vaginal, systemic), other fungal infections (esp tinea, pityriasis).

Caution: susceptibility to ↑QTc, L/R/P/B.

SE: GI upset, **hypersensitivity** (can ⇒ angioedema, TEN, SJS, anaphylaxis: if develops rash, stop drug or monitor closely), **hepato-toxicity**, headache. Rarely blood/metabolic (↑lipids, ↓K$^+$) disorders, dizziness, seizures, alopecia.

Monitor: LFTs; stop drug if features of liver disease develop.

Interactions: ↓**P450** ∴ many; most importantly, ↑s fx of theophyl-lines, ciclosporin, phenytoin and tacrolimus. Also ↓ clopidogrel fx. **W** + .

Dose: 50–400 mg/day po or iv according to indication[SPC/BNF].
NB: ↓dose in RF.

FLUDROCORTISONE

Mineralocorticoid (also has glucocorticoid actions).

Use: adrenocortical deficiency, esp Addison's disease[1].

CI/Caution/Interactions: See Prednisolone.

SE: H$_2$O/Na$^+$ retention, ↓K$^+$ (monitor U&Es). Also can ⇒ immunosuppression (and other SEs of corticosteroids; see p. 227).

Dose: 50–300 microgram/day po[1].

FLUMAZENIL

Benzodiazepine antagonist (competitive).

Use: benzodiazepine OD/toxicity (only if respiratory depression and ventilatory support not immediately available).

CI: life-threatening conditions controlled by benzodiazepines (e.g. ↑ICP, status epilepticus).

Caution: mixed ODs (esp TCAs), benzodiazepine dependence (may ⇒ withdrawal fx; see p. 229), Hx of panic disorder (can ⇒ relapse), head injury, epileptics on long-term benzodiazepine Rx (may ⇒ fits), L/P/B/E.

SE: N&V, dizziness, flushing, rebound anxiety/agitation, transient ↑BP/HR. Very rarely anaphylaxis.

Dose: initially 200 microgram iv over 15 sec, then, if required, further doses of 100 microgram at 1 min intervals. *Max total dose 1 mg (2 mg in ITU)*. Can also give as ivi at 100–400 microgram/h adjusting to response. NB: see p. 266 for Rx of acute OD.

NB: short $t_{1/2}$ (40–80 min); observe closely after Rx and consider further doses or ivi (at 0.1–0.4 mg/h adjusted to response).

> 🔹 *Flumazenil is not recommended as a diagnostic test and should not be given routinely in overdoses as risk of inducing:*
>
> - fits (esp if epileptic, or if co-ingested drugs that predispose to fits)
> - withdrawal syndrome (if habituated to benzodiazepines)
> - arrhythmias (esp if co-ingested TCA or amphetamine-like drug).
>
> If in any doubt get senior opinion and exclude habituation to benzodiazepines and get ECG before giving unless life-threatening respiratory depression and benzodiazepine known to be cause ☠.

FLUOXETINE/PROZAC

SSRI antidepressant: long $t_{1/2}$ compared with others*.

Use: depression[1], other Ψ disorders (inc bulimia[2], OCD[3]).

CI: active mania.

Caution: epilepsy, receiving ECT, Hx of mania or bleeding disorder (esp GI), heart disease, DM†, glaucoma (angle closure), ↑risk of bleeding, age < 18 yrs **L/R/H/P/B/E**.

Class SEs: GI upset, ↓Wt, insomnia**, agitation**, headache, hypersensitivity. Can ⇒ withdrawal fx when stopped (see p. 235) ∴ *stop slowly*; more important for SSRIs with ↓$t_{1/2}$*. Rarely extrapyramidal (see p. 236) and antimuscarinic fx (see p. 233), sexual dysfunction, convulsions, ↓Na^+ (inc SIADH), blood disorders, GI bleed, serotonin syndrome (see p. 236) and suicidal thoughts/behaviour.

Specific SEs: rarely hypoglycaemia†, vasculitis (rash may be 1st sign).

Warn: can ↓performance at skilled tasks (inc driving). Don't stop suddenly (not as important as for other SSRIs).

Interactions: ↓P450 ∴ many, but most importantly ↑s levels of TCAs, benzodiazepines, clozapine and haloperidol. ↑s lithium toxicity and ⇒ HTN and ↑CNS fx with sele-/rasa-giline (and other

dopaminergics). ↑risk of CNS toxicity with drugs that ↑5HT (e.g. tramadol, sibutramine, sumatriptan, St John's wort). ↑risk of bleeding with aspirin and NSAIDs. Levels ↑by ritonavir. Antagonises anti-epileptics (but ↑s levels of carbamazepine and phenytoin). Avoid with artemether/lumefantrine and tamoxifen. ☠ *Never give with, or*
≤2 wks after, MAOIs☠. (Mild **W** + .)
Dose: initially 20 mg[1,3] (↑to max 60 mg) od; 60 mg od[2] – give mane as can ↓sleep**.
NB: ↓dose in LF.

FLUTICASONE/FLIXOTIDE (various delivery devices available[BNF])
Inhaled corticosteroid for asthma: see Beclometasone.
Dose: 100–2000 microgram/day inh (or 0.5–2 mg bd as nebs).

1 microgram equivalent to 2 microgram of beclometasone or budesonide.

FOLIC ACID (= FOLATE)

Vitamin: building block of nucleic acids. Essential co-factor for DNA synthesis ⇒ normal erythropoiesis.
Use: megaloblastic ↓Hb Rx/Px if haemolysis/dialysis[1] (or GI malab-sorption where ↑doses may be needed), Px against neural-tube dfx in pregnancy[2] (esp if on antiepileptics), Px of mucositis and GI upset if on methotrexate[3].
CI: malignancy (unless megaloblastic ↓Hb due to ↓folate is an important complication).
Caution: undiagnosed megaloblastic ↓Hb (i.e. ↓B₁₂, as found in pernicious anaemia) – never give alone if *B_{12} deficiency as can precipitate subacute combined degeneration of spinal cord.*
SE: GI disturbance (rare).
Dose: 5 mg od[1] (in maintenance, ↓frequency of dose, often to wkly); 400 microgram od from before conception until wk 12 of pregnancy[2] (unless mother has neural-tube defect herself or has previously had a child with a neural-tube defect, when 5 mg od needed); 5 mg once wkly[3].

FOMEPIZOLE Antidote for toxic alcohols.

▼ FONDAPARINUX/ARIXTRA

Anticoagulant; activated factor X inhibitor.
Use: ACS (UA, NSTEMI or STEMI), Px of VTE, Rx of DVT/PE.
CI: active bleeding, bacterial endocarditis.
Caution: bleeding disorders, active PU, other drugs that ↑risk of
bleeding, recent intracranial haemorrhage, recent brain/ophthalmic/
spinal surgery, spinal/epidural anaesthesia (avoid Rx doses), Wt <50
kg. **R** (avoid or ↓dose according to indication and creatinine
clearance[SPC/BNF]), **L/P/B/E.**
SE: bleeding, ↓Hb, ↓(or ↑)Pt, coagulopathy, purpura, oedema, LFT
Δs, GI upset. Rarely ↓K⁺, ↓BP, hypersensitivity.
Dose: UA/NSTEMI/Px of VTE 2.5 mg sc od (start 6-h post-op);
STEMI 2.5 mg iv/ivi od for 1st day then sc; Rx of PE/DVT by
Wt (<50 kg = 5 mg sc od, 50–100 kg = 7.5 mg sc od, >100 kg = 10
mg sc od). NB: Length of Rx depends on indication[SPC/BNF], timing of
doses post-op critical if Wt <50 kg or elderly. **Consider** ↓dose in RF.

Specialist use only: get senior advice or contact on-call cardiology/
haematology.

FORMOTEROL (= EFORMOTEROL)/FORADIL, OXIS

Long-acting β₂ agonist 'LABA'; as Salmeterol plus **L.**
Dose: 6–48 microgram daily (mostly bd regime)[SPC/BNF] inh (min/max
doses vary with preparations[SPC/BNF]).

FOSPHENYTOIN

Antiepileptic: prodrug of phenytoin; allows safer rapid loading.
Use: epilepsy (esp 'status' & seizures assoc with neurosurgery/head
injury).
CI/Caution/SE/Monitor/Warn/Interactions: as phenytoin, but
↓SEs (esp ↓arrhythmias and 'purple glove syndrome').
Dose: as phenytoin, but prescribe as 'phenytoin sodium equivalent'
and note ☠fosphenytoin 1.5 mg = phenytoin 1 mg☠.
NB: consider ↓dose in LF or RF.

FOSTAIR

Combination asthma inhaler: each puff contains 100 microgram beclomethasone (steroid) + 6 microgram formoterol (long-acting β_2-agonist) in a metered dose inhaler.

Dose: 1–2 puffs bd inh.

▼ FRAGMIN see ▼ Dalteparin; low-molecular-weight heparin.

FRUMIL see Co-amilofruse; tablets are 5/40 (5 mg amiloride + 40 mg furosemide) unless stated as LS (2.5/20) or FORTE (10/80).

FRUSEMIDE now called Furosemide.

FUROSEMIDE (previously Frusemide).

Loop diuretic: inhibits Na^+/K^+ pump in ascending loop of Henle $\Rightarrow$ ↓resorption and ∴ ↑loss of $Na^+/K^+/Cl/H_2O$.

Use: LVF (esp in acute pulmonary oedema, but also in chronic LVF/ CCF or as Px during blood transfusion), resistant HTN (*for advice on stepped HTN Mx see p. 182*), oliguria secondary to AKI (after correcting hypovolaemia first).

CI: ↓↓K^+, ↓Na^+, cirrhosis (if precomatose), **R** (if anuria).

Caution: ↓BP, ↑prostate, porphyria, diabetes, **L/P/B**.

SE: ↓BP (inc postural), ↓K^+, ↓Na^+, ↓Ca^{2+}, ↓Mg^{2+}, ↓Cl alkalosis. Also ↑**urate/gout**, GI upset, ↑glucose/impaired glucose tolerance, ↑cholesterol/TGs (temporary). Rarely **BM suppression** (stop drug), RF, skin reactions, pancreatitis, tinnitus/deafness (if ↑doses or RF: reversible).

Interactions: ↑s toxicity of digoxin, flecanide, solatol, NSAIDs, vancomycin, gentamicin and lithium. ↓s fx of antidiabetics. NSAIDs may ↓diuretic response.

Monitor: U&Es; if ↓K^+, add po K^+ supplements/K^+-sparing diuretic or change to combination tablet (e.g. co-amilofruse).

Dose: usually 20–80 mg po/im/iv daily in divided doses. ↑doses used in acute LVF (see p. 243) and oliguria. If HF or RF, ivi (max 4 mg/min) can $\Rightarrow$ smoother control of fluid balance$^{SPC/BNF}$. For blood transfusions, a rough guide is to give 20 mg with every unit if *existing*

LVF, and with every 2nd unit if *at risk of LVF.* **NB: may need ↑dose in RF.**

Give iv if severe oedema: as bowel oedema ⇒ ↓po absorption.

FUSIDIC ACID/FUCIDIN

Antibiotic; good bone penetration and activity against *S. aureus*.
Use: osteomyelitis, endocarditis (2° to penicillin-resistant staphylococci) – needs 2nd antibiotic to prevent resistance.
Caution: biliary disease or obstruction (⇒ ↓elimination), L/P/B.
SE: GI upset, hepatitis*. Rarely: skin/blood disorders, AKI.
Monitor: LFTs* (esp if chronic Rx, ↑doses or LF).
Dose: 500 mg tds po (equivalent to 750 mg tds if using suspension) – in severe infection to ↑1 g tds po; 500 mg tds iv (6–7 mg/kg tds if Wt <50 kg). **NB: ↓dose in LF.**

FUSIDIC ACID 1% EYE DROPS/FUCITHALMIC

Topical antibiotic (esp vs. *Staphylococcus*); commonly used for blepharitis.
Dose: 1 drop bd.

FYBOGEL

Laxative: bulking agent (ispaghula husk) for constipation (inc IBS).
CI: ↓swallow, GI obstruction, faecal impaction, colonic atony.
Dose: 1 sachet or 10 ml bd after meals with water.

GABAPENTIN

Antiepileptic: similar structure to GABA but mechanism of action is different from drugs affecting GABA receptors.
Use: neuropathic pain, epilepsy (adjunctive Rx of partial seizures ± 2° generalisation).
Caution: Hx of psychosis or DM, R/P/B/E.
SE: fatigue/somnolence, dizziness, cerebellar fx (esp ataxia; see p. 236), dipl-/ambly-opia, headache, rhinitis. Rarely ↓WCC, GI upset, arthra-/my-algia, skin reactions, suicidal ideation.
Interactions: fx ↓by antidepressants and antimalarials (esp mefloquine).

Dose: initially 300 mg od, ↑ing by 300 mg/day to max 3.6 g daily in 3 divided doses (*NB: stop drug over ≥1 wk*). **NB: ↓dose in RF.**

Can give false-positive urinary dipstick results for proteinuria.

GASTROCOTE Compound alginate for acid reflux.

Dose: 5–15 ml or 1–2 tablets after meals and at bedtime (NB: 2.13 mmol Na^+/5 ml and 1 mmol Na^+/tablet).

GAVISCON (ADVANCE) Alginate raft-forming oral suspension for acid reflux.
Dose: 5–10 ml or 1–2 tablets after meals and at bedtime (NB: 2.3 mmol Na^+ and 1 mmol K^+/5 ml and 2.25 mmol Na^+ and 1 mmol K^+/tablet).

Ensure good hydration, esp if elderly, GI narrowing or ↓GI motility.

GELOFUSINE

Colloid plasma substitute (gelatin-based) for iv fluid resuscitation (see p. 222). 1 l contains 154 mmol Na^+(but no K^+).

GENTAMICIN

Aminoglycoside: broad-spectrum 'cidal' antibiotic; inhibs ribosomal 30S subunit. Good Gram-negative aerobe/staphylococci cover; other organisms often need concurrent penicillin ± metronidazole.
Use: severe infections, esp sepsis, meningitis, endocarditis. Also pyelonephritis/prostatitis, biliary tract infections, pneumonia.
CI: MG*.
Caution: obesity, R/P/B/E.
SE: **ototoxic, nephrotoxic** (dose- and Rx length-dependent), **hypersensitivity**, rash. Rarely AAC, N&V, seizures, encephalopathy, blood disorders, myasthenia-like syndrome* (at ↑doses; reversible), ↓ Mg^{2+} (if prolonged Rx).
Monitor: serum levels** after 3 or 4 doses (earlier if RF).
Interactions: fx (esp toxicity) ↑by loop diuretics (esp **furosemide**), cephalosporins, vancomycin, amphotericin, ciclosporin, tacrolimus and cytotoxics; if these drugs must be given, space doses as far from

time of gentamicin dose as possible. ↑s fx of muscle relaxants and anticholinesterases. **W** + .

Dose: once daily regimen: initially 5–7 mg/kg ivi adjusting to levels (NB: consult local protocol; od regimen not suitable if endocarditis, >20% total body surface burns or creatinine clearance <20 ml/min).

Multiple daily regimen: 3–5 mg/kg/day in 3 divided doses im/iv/ivi (if endocarditis give 1 mg/kg tds iv).

NB: ↓doses if RF (and consider if elderly or ↑↑BMI), otherwise adjust according to serum levels*: call microbiology department if unsure.

**Gentamicin levels: Measure peak at 1 h post-dose (ideally = 5–10 mg/l) and trough immediately predose (ideally ≤2 mg/l). Halve ideal peak levels if for endocarditis. If levels high, can ↑*spacing* of doses (as well as ↓ing *amount* of dose); as ⇒↑risk of ototoxicity, monitor auditory/vestibular function.
*NB: od regimens usually only require **pre-dose** level.*

GLIBENCLAMIDE

Oral antidiabetic (long-acting sulphonylurea): ↑s pancreatic insulin release – stimulates β islet cell receptors (and inhibits gluconeogenesis).

Use: type 2 DM; requires endogenous insulin to work. Not recommended for obese* (use metformin) or elderly** (use short-acting preparations, e.g. gliclazide).

CI: ketoacidosis, acute porphyria, **L/R** (if either severe, otherwise caution), **P/B**.

Caution: may need to replace with insulin during intercurrent illness/surgery, porphyria, **E**.

SE: hypoglycaemia (esp in elderly**), **GI upset**, ↑Wt*. Rarely hypersensitivity (inc skin) reactions, blood disorders, hepatotoxicity and transient visual Δs (esp initially).

Interactions: fx ↑d by chloramphenicol, sulphonamides (inc co-trimoxazole), sulfinpyrazone, antifungals (esp flu-/mic-onazole), warfarin, fibrates and NSAIDs. Levels ↓by rifampicin/rifabutin. ↑Risk of hepatotoxicity with bosentan.

Dose: initially 5 mg mane (with food), ↑ing as necessary (max 15 mg/day).

NB: ↓dose in severe LF.

GLICLAZIDE

Oral antidiabetic (short-acting sulphonylurea).

Use/CI/Caution/SE/Interactions: as glibenclamide, but shorter action* and hepatic metabolism** mean ↓d risk of hypoglycaemia (esp in elderly* and RF**).

Dose: initially 40–80 mg mane (with food), ↑ing as necessary (max 320 mg/day). MR tablets available (Diamicron MR) of which 30 mg has equivalent effect to 80 mg of normal release (dose initially is 30 mg od, ↑ing if necessary to max 120 mg od). **NB: ↓dose in RF or severe LF.**

GLIMEPIRIDE

Oral antidiabetic (short-acting sulphonylurea).

Use/CI/Caution/SE/Interactions: as gliclazide, plus manufacturer recommends monitoring of FBC and LFTs. CI in severe LF. May need to substitute with insulin; seek specialist advice.

Dose: initially 1 mg mane (with food), ↑ing as necessary (max 6 mg/day).

GLIPIZIDE

Oral antidiabetic (short-acting sulphonylurea).

Use/CI/Caution/SE/Interactions: as gliclazide, plus avoid if both L and R.

Dose: initially 2.5–5.0 mg mane (with food), ↑ing as necessary (max single dose 15 mg; max daily dose 20 mg).

NB: ↓dose in severe LF and RF.

GLUCAGON

Polypeptide hormone: ↑s hepatic glycogen conversion to glucose.

Use: hypoglycaemia: if acute and severe, esp if no iv access or if 2° to xs insulin (see p. 256).

CI: phaeo.

Caution: glucagonomas/insulinomas. Will not work if hypoglycaemia is chronic (inc starvation) or $2°$ to adrenal insufficiency.
SE: N&V&D, $\downarrow$BP, $\downarrow K^+$, rarely hypersensitivity, **W** + .
Dose: 1 mg (= 1 unit) **im** (or sc/iv)$^{SPC/BNF}$.

Often stocked in cardiac arrest ('crash') trolleys.

GLYCEROL (= GLYCERIN) SUPPOSITORIES

Rectal irritant bowel stimulant.
Use: constipation: 1st-line suppository if oral methods such as lactulose and senna fail.
Dose: 1–2 pr prn.

GLYCERYL TRINITRATE see GTN.

GRANISETRON

Antiemetic: $5HT_3$ antagonist.
Use: N&V; see Ondansetron.
Caution: GI obstruction (inc subacute), $\uparrow$QTc, **P/B**.
SE: constipation (or diarrhoea), **headache**, sedation, fatigue, dizziness. Rarely seizures, chest pain, $\downarrow$BP, Δ LFTs, rash, hypersensitivity.
Dose: 1 mg bd or 2 mg od po/iv/ivi for non-specialist use. 2–3 mg loading doses often given before chemotherapy$^{SPC/BNF}$ (max 9 mg/24 h).

GTN (= GLYCERYL TRINITRATE)

Nitrate: $\Rightarrow$ coronary artery + systemic vein dilation $\Rightarrow$ $\uparrow O_2$ supply to myocardium and $\downarrow$preload, $\therefore$ $\downarrow O_2$ demand of myocardium.
Use: Angina, LVF.
CI: $\downarrow$BP, $\downarrow\downarrow$Hb, aortic/mitral stenosis, constrictive pericarditis, tamponade, HOCM, glaucoma (closed-angle), hypovolaemia, $\uparrow$ICP.
Caution: recent MI, $\downarrow T_4$, hypothermia, head trauma, cerebral haemorrhage, malnutrition, **L/R** (if either severe).
SE: $\downarrow$BP (inc postural), **headache**, dizziness, flushing, $\uparrow$HR.

Interactions: ☠ sildenafil, tadalafil and vardenafil (are CI as ⇒ ↓↓BP). ☠. ↓s fx of heparins (if given iv).

Warn: may develop tolerance with ↓therapeutic effect (esp if long-term transdermal patch use) and don't stop abruptly.

Dose: 2 sprays or tablets sl prn (also available as transdermal SR patches[SPC/BNF]). For acute MI/LVF: 10–200 microgram/min ivi, titrating to clinical response and BP (see p. 240).

HALOPERIDOL

Butyrophenone ('typical') antipsychotic: dopamine antagonist ($D_{2 \text{ and } 3}$ > $D_{1 \text{ and } 4}$). Also blocks serotonin ($5HT_{2A}$), histamine (H_1), adrenergic ($\alpha_{1>2}$) and muscarinic receptors, causing many SEs.

Use: acute sedation[1] (e.g. agitation and behavioural disturbance), schizophrenia/bipolar disorder[2], N&V[3].

CI/Caution/SE: as chlorpromazine, but ⇒ ↑incidence of **extrapyramidal fx** (see p. 236), although ⇒ ↓sedation, ↓skin reactions, ↓antimuscarinic fx, ↓BP fx, but can ⇒ hypoglycaemia and SIADH. Also risk of CNS toxicity with lithium.

Interactions: metab by P450 [many, but most importantly: levels ↑by fluoxetine, venlafaxine, quinidine, buspirone and ritonavir]. Levels ↓by carbamazepine, phenytoin, rifampicin. ↑risk of arrhythmias with amiodarone and ↓s fx of anticonvulsants.

Dose: 1.5–5.0 mg bd/tds po (max 30 mg/day)[1,2]; 2–10 mg im/iv 4–8-hrly (max 18 mg/day)[1,2]; 0.5–2.0 mg tds im/sc/iv[3]. Also used im as a 4-wkly 'depot'[2] if concerns over compliance. NB: ↓**dose in severe RF or elderly.**

Start at bottom of dose range if naive to antipsychotics, esp if elderly. See p. 227 for advice on acute sedation.

HARTMANN'S SOLUTION

Compound sodium lactate iv fluid. GIFTASUP guidelines recommend this over 0.9% NaCl in surgical patients for resuscitation or fluid replacement unless vomiting/gastric losses. 1 l contains 5 mmol K^+, 2 mmol Ca^{2+}, 29 mmol HCO_3, 131 mmol Na^+, 111 mmol Cl^-.

HEPARIN, standard/unfractionated (NB: $\neq$ LMWHs).

iv (and rarely sc) anticoagulant: potentiates protease inhibitor antithrombin III, which inactivates thrombin. Also inhibits factors IXa/Xa/XIa/XIIa.

Use: anticoagulation if needs to be immediate or quickly reversible (only as inpatient); DVT/PE Rx/Px (inc preoperative), MI/unstable angina Rx/Px, extracorporeal circuits (esp haemodialysis, cardiopulmonary bypass).

CI: haemorrhagic disorders (inc haemophilia), ↓Pt (inc Hx of HIT*), severe HTN, PU, acute bacterial endocarditis, recent cerebral haemorrhage or major surgery/trauma to eye/brain/spinal cord, epidural/spinal anaesthesia (but can give Px doses), **L** (if severe, esp if oesophageal varices).

Caution: ↑K$^+$**, R/P/E.

SE: haemorrhage, ↓Pt* (HIT*), **hypersensitivity** (inc anaphylaxis, urticaria, angioedema), ↑K$^+$** (inhibits aldosterone: ↑risk if DM, CRF, acidosis or on K$^+$-sparing drugs), osteoporosis (if prolonged Rx).

Monitor: FBC* if >5 days Rx, U&E** if > 7 days Rx.

Interactions: fx may ↓by GTN ivi. NSAIDs ⇒ ↑bleeding risk.

Dose: see p. 212 (inc dose-adjustment advice).

☠HIT* Heparin Induced Thrombocytopenia: immune mediated ∴ delayed onset – ↑risk if Rx for >5 days (see p. 212)☠.

HUMALOG see Insulin lispro; short-acting recombinant insulin. Also available as biphasic preparations (Mix 25, Mix 50), are combined with longer-acting isophane suspension.

HUMULIN Recombinant insulin available in various forms:

1 HUMULIN S soluble, short-acting for iv/acute use.

2 HUMULIN I isophane (combined with protamine), long-acting.

3 HUMULIN M 'biphasic' preparations, combination of short-acting (S) and long-acting (I) forms to give smoother control throughout the day. Numbers denote 1/10% of soluble insulin (i.e. M3 = 30% soluble insulin).

HYDRALAZINE

Antihypertensive: vasodilates smooth muscle (arteries > veins).
Use: HTN[1] (inc severe[2], esp if RF or pregnancy), HF[3]. *For advice on HTN Mx see p. 182.*
CI: severe ↑HR, myocardial insufficiency (2° to mechanical obstruction, e.g. aortic/mitral stenosis or constrictive pericarditis), cor pulmonale, dissecting aortic aneurysm, SLE*, porphyria, **H** (if 'high output', e.g. ↑T_4).
Caution: IHD, cerebrovascular disease, L/R/P/B.
SE: (*all SEs ↓if dose 100 mg/day*) ↑HR, GI upset, **headache, lupus-like syndrome*** (watch for unexplained ↓Wt, arthritis, ill health – measure ANA* and dipstick urine for protein if on high doses/clinical suspicion). Also fluid retention (↓d if used with diuretics), palpitations, dizziness, flushing, ↓BP (even at low doses), blood disorders, arthr-/my-algia, rash and can worsen IHD.
Dose: 25–50 mg bd po[1]; 5–10 mg iv[2] (can be repeated after 20–30 min) or 50–300 microgram/min ivi[2]; 25–75 mg tds/qds po[3].
NB: ↓dose if LF or RF.

HYDROCORTISONE BUTYRATE CREAM (0.1%)

Potent-strength topical corticosteroid. NB: much stronger than 'standard' (i.e. non-butyrate) hydrocortisone cream; see below!

HYDROCORTISONE CREAM/OINTMENT (1%)

Mild-strength topical corticosteroid (rarely used as weaker 0.5%, 0.25% and 0.1% preparations).
Use: inflammatory skin conditions, in particular eczema.
CI: untreated infection, rosacea, acne.
SE: rare compared to more potent steroids: skin atrophy, worsening of infections, acne.
Dose: apply thinly 1 or 2 times per day.

HYDROCORTISONE iv/po

Glucocorticoid (with significant mineralocorticoid activity).

infusion[2] (see p. 189 for use in palliative care); 300 microgram bd po[3] (can ↑to tds).

Don't confuse with hyoscine *butylbromide*: different fx and doses!

HYPROMELLOSE 0.3% EYE DROPS

Artificial tears for treatment of dry eyes.
Dose: 1 drop prn, max 4–6 times/day unless preservative free drops.

IBUGEL Ibuprofen topical gel, for musculoskeletal pain.

IBUPROFEN

Mild-moderate strength NSAID. Non-selective COX inhibitor; analgesic, anti-inflammatory and antipyrexial[†] properties.
Use: mild/moderate pain[1] (inc musculoskeletal, headache, migraine, dysmenorrhoea, dental, post-op; not 1st choice for gout/RA as ↓anti-inflammatory fx compared to other NSAIDs), mild local inflammation[2].
CI: Hx of hypersensitivity to aspirin or any other NSAID (inc asthma/angioedema/urticaria/rhinitis). **Active/Hx of PU/GI bleeding/perforation, L/R/H** (if any of these 3 are severe)/**P** (3rd trimester).
Caution: Asthma, allergic disorders, uncontrolled HTN, IHD, PVD, cerebrovascular disease, cardiovascular risk factors, connective tissue disorders, coagulopathy, IBD. *Can mask signs of infection[†]*. **L/R/H/P** (1st/2nd trimester: preferably avoid)/**B/E**.
SE: GI upset/bleeding/PU (*less than other NSAIDs*). AKI, hypersensitivity reactions (esp bronchospasm and skin reactions, inc, very rarely, SJS/TEN), fluid retention/oedema, headache, dizziness, nervousness, depression, drowsiness, insomnia, tinnitus, photosensitivity, haematuria. >1.2 g/day ⇒ small ↑risk thrombotic events. Reversible ↓female fertility if long-term use. Very rarely, blood disorders, ↑BP, ↑K^+.
Interactions: ↑risk GI bleeding with aspirin, clopidogrel, anticoagulants, corticosteroids, SSRIs, venlafaxine and erlotinib. ↑s (toxic) fx of digoxin, quinolones, lithium, phenytoin, baclofen, methotrexate, AZT and sulphonylureas. ↑risk of RF with ACE-i, ARB, diuretics, tacrolimus and ciclosporin. ↑risk ↑K^+ with K-sparing diuretics and

aldosterone antagonists. ↓s fx of antihypertensives and diuretics.
↑levels with ritonavir and triazoles. Mild **W +** .
Dose: initially 300–400 mg tds po[1] (max 2.4 g/day); topically as gel[2].
NB: Avoid/↓dose in RF & consider gastroprotective Rx.

INDAPAMIDE

Thiazide derivative diuretic; see Bendroflumethiazide.
Use: HTN (*for advice on stepped HTN Mx see p. 182*).
CI: Hx of sulphonamide derivative allergy, ↓K$^+$, ↓Na$^+$, ↑Ca^{2+}, **L/R**
(if either severe).
Caution: ↑PTH (stop if ↑Ca^{2+}), ↑aldosterone, gout, porphyria,
R/P/B/E.
SE: as bendroflumethiazide, but reportedly fewer metabolic disturbances (esp less hyperglycaemia).
Monitor: U&Es, urate.
Interactions: ↑s lithium levels and toxicity of digoxin (if ⇒ ↓K$^+$).
Dose: 2.5 mg od mane (or 1.5 mg od of SR preparation).

INDOMETACIN

High-strength NSAID; non-selective COX inhibitor.
Use: musculoskeletal pain[1], esp RA, ankylosing spondylitis, OA; acute
gout[2]; dysmenorrhoea[3]. Use limited by SEs*. Specialist uses: PDA
closure, premature labour[SPC/BNF].
CI/Caution/SE/Interactions: as ibuprofen, but ↑incidence of SEs*,
inc PU/GI bleeds, thrombotic events, GI upset and headache. Lightheadedness (impairing driving) is common. Rarely: Ψ disturbances,
convulsions, syncope, blood disorders, ↑CBG, peripheral neuropathy,
optic neuritis, intestinal strictures; pr doses may ⇒ rectal irritation/
bleeding. Caution in epilepsy, Parkinsonism & Ψ disturbance.
Probenecid ⇒ ↑serum levels. ↑risk of AKI with triamterene: avoid.
Possible severe drowsiness with haloperidol. No known interaction
with baclofen or triazoles. Mild **W +** .
Dose: 25–50 mg max qds po or 100 mg max bd pr[1]. 150–200 mg/day
in divided doses, ↓ing dose once pain under control[2]. 75 mg/day in
divided doses[3]. MR preparations available[SPC/BNF].

NB: Avoid/↓dose in RF & consider gastroprotective Rx.

INFLIXIMAB/REMICADE

Monoclonal Ab against TNF-α (inflammatory cytokine).

Use: Crohn's/UC[NICE], RA[NICE], psoriasis (for skin or arthritis)[NICE] or ankylosing spondylitis[NICE].

CI: TB or other severe infections, **H** (unless mild when only caution), **P/B**.

Caution: infections, demyelinating CNS disorders, **L/R**.

SE: severe infections, TB (inc extrapulmonary), CCF (exac of), CNS demyelination. Also GI upset, 'flu-like symptoms, cough, fatigue, headache, ↑incidence of hypersensitivity (esp transfusion) reactions.

Dose: specialist use only. Often prescribed concurrently with methotrexate.

INSULATARD Long-acting (isophane) insulin, either recombinant human or porcine/bovine.

INSULIN see p. 202 for different types and prescribing advice.

INTEGRILIN see Eptifibatide; anti-Pt agent for IHD.

IODINE and IODIDE see Lugol's solution; used for ↑↑T_4.

IPOCOL see Mesalazine; 'new' aminosalicylate for UC, with ↓SEs.

IPRATROPIUM

Inh muscarinic antagonist; bronchodilator and ↓s bronchial secretions.

Use: chronic[1] and acute[2] bronchospasm (COPD > asthma). Rarely used topically for rhinitis.

SE: antimuscarinic fx (see p. 233), usually minimal.

Caution: glaucoma (angle closure only; protect patient's eyes from drug, esp if giving nebs: use tight-fitting mask), bladder outflow obstruction (e.g. ↑prostate), **P/B**.

Dose: 20–40 microgram tds/qds inh[1] (max 80 microgram qds); 250–500 microgram qds neb[2] (↑ing up to 4-hrly if severe).

IRBESARTAN/APROVEL

Angiotensin II antagonist.

Use: HTN (*for advice on stepped HTN Mx see p. 182*), type 2 DM nephropathy.

CI: **P/B**.

Caution/SE/Interactions: see Losartan.

Dose: initially 150 mg od, ↑ing to 300 mg od if required (halve initial dose if age >75 years or on haemodialysis).

IRON TABLETS see Ferrous sulphate/fumarate/gluconate.

ISMN see Isosorbide mononitrate.

ISMO see Isosorbide mononitrate.

ISONIAZID

Antituberculous antibiotic; 'static'.

Use: TB (see p. 175).

CI: drug-induced liver disease.

Caution: Hx of psychosis/epilepsy/porphyria or if ↑d risk of neuropathy[†] (e.g. DM, alcohol abuse, CRF, malnutrition, HIV: give pyridoxine 10–20 mg od as Px), porphyria, **L/R/P/B**.

SE: optic neuritis, **peripheral neuropathy**[†], **hepatitis**[*], rash, gynaeco-mastia, GI upset. Rarely lupus, blood disorders (inc rarely agranulo-cytosis[**]), hypersensitivity, convulsions, psychosis.

Warn: patient of symptoms of liver disease and to seek medical help if they occur.

Monitor: LFTs[*], FBC[**].

Interactions: ↓**P450** ∴ many, but most importantly ↑s levels of carbamazepine, phenytoin, ethosuximide and benzodiazepines **W** + .

Dose: by weight[SPC/BNF] or as combination preparation (see p. 175). Take on empty stomach (≥30 min before or ≥ 2 h after meal).

Acetylator-dependent metabolism: if slow acetylator ⇒ ↑risk of SEs.

ISOSORBIDE MONONITRATE (ISMN)

Nitrate; as GTN, but po rather than sl delivery.
Use/Cl/Caution/SE/Interactions: as GTN, but ⇒ ↓headache.
Dose: 10–40 mg bd/tds po (od MR preparations available[SPC/BNF]).

ISTIN see Amlodipine; Ca^{2+} channel blocker for HTN/IHD.

ITRACONAZOLE/SPORANOX

Triazole antifungal: needs acidic pH for good po absorption*.
Use: fungal infections (candida, tinea, cryptococcus, aspergillosis, histoplasmosis, onychomycosis, pityriasis versicolor).
Caution: risk of HF: Hx of cardiac disease or if on negative inotropic drugs (risk ↑s with dose, length of Rx and age), **L/R/P/B**.
SE: HF, hepatotoxicity**, GI upset, headache, dizziness, peripheral neuropathy (if occurs, stop drug), cholestasis, menstrual Δs, skin reactions (inc angioedema, SJS). With prolonged Rx can ⇒ ↓K^+, oedema, hair loss.
Monitor: LFTs** if Rx >1 month or Hx of (or develop clinical features of) liver disease: stop drug if become abnormal.
Interactions: ↓**P450** ∴ many; most importantly ↑s risk of **myopathy with statins** (avoid together) and ↑s risk of **HF with negative inotropes** (esp Ca^{2+} blockers). ↑s fx of 🚗 **midazolam, quinidine, pimozide** 🚗, ciclosporin, digoxin, indinavir and siro-/tacro-limus. fx ↓d by rifampicin, phenytoin and **antacids***, **W +**.
Dose: dependent on indication[SPC/BNF]. *Take capsules with food (or liquid on empty stomach).* NB: consider ↓dose in LF.

▼ IVABRADINE/PROCORALAN

↓s HR by selective cardiac pacemaker I_f channel current blockade ⇒ ↓SAN myocyte Na^+ and K^+ entry.
Use: angina (if sinus rhythm and β-blockers CI/not tolerated).
CI: severe ↓HR (<60bpm) or ↓BP, cardiogenic shock, ACS (inc acute MI), acute CVA, 2nd or 3rd degree HB, SSS, pacemaker dependent, SAN block congenital ↑QT syndrome, strong **P450 3A4** inhibitors**, **L**(if severe)/**H**(if moderate/severe)/**P/B**.

Caution: retinitis pigmentosa, galactose intolerance*/Lapp lactase deficiency*/glucose-galactose malabsorption*, R/E.

SE: visual Δs (esp luminous phenomena*), ↓HR, HB, ectopics, VF, headaches, dizziness. Less commonly GI upset, cramps, dyspnoea, ↑EØ, ↑uric acid, ↓GFR.

Warn: tablets contain lactose*, may ↓vision if night driving/using machinery with rapid light intensity Δs.

Monitor: HR (maintain resting ventricular rate > 50 bpm) and rhythm, BP.

Interactions: ☠ metab by P450 3A4; inhibitors ↑levels and strong inhibitors** (clari-/ery-/josa-/teli-thromycin, itra-/keto-cona-zole, nelfi-/rito-navir, nefazodone) are CI but ↓doses can be given with fluconazole. Inducers ↓levels (inc rifampicin, barbiturates, phenytoin, St John's wort). Levels also ↑by diltiazem and verapamil. ↑risk of VF with drugs that ↑QTc (inc amiodarone, disopyramide, mefloquine, pentamidine, pimozide, sertindole, sotalol)☠.

Dose: initially 5 mg bd po; ↑ing if required after 3–4 wks to max 7.5 mg bd po.

NB: consider ↓dose if not tolerated, elderly or severe RF$^{SPC/BNF}$.

KAY-CEE-L

KCl syrup (1 mmol/ml) for ↓K$^+$; see Sando-K.

Dose: according to serum K$^+$: average 25–50 ml/day in divided doses if diet normal. Caution if taking other drugs that ↑K$^+$.

NB: ↓dose if RF.

KETOCONAZOLE/NIZORAL

Imidazole antifungal: good po absorption.

Use: fungal infection Rx (if systemic, severe or resistant to topical Rx) and Px if immunosuppression; use limited (due to hepatotoxicity) to dermatophytosis, *Malassezia* folliculitis and cutaneous or oro-pharyngeal candidosis and only when topical and oral agents can't be used.

CI: L/P/B.

Caution: porphyria.

SE: hepatitis*, **GI upset**, **skin reactions** (rash, urticaria, pruritus, photosensitivity, rarely angioedema), **gynaecomastia**, blood disorders, paraesthesia, dizziness, photophobia.

Monitor: LFTs*, esp if Rx >14 days.

Warn: seek urgent medical attention if signs of LF (explain symptoms to patient).

Interactions: ↓P450 ∴ many; most importantly, ↑s risk of **myopathy with statins** (avoid together). ↑s fx of 💀 **midazolam, quinidine, pimozide** 💀, vardenafil, eplerenone, cilostazol, reboxetine, aripiprazole, sertindole, felodipine, ergot alkaloids, antidiabetics, buprenorphine, artemether/lumefantrine, indi-/rito-navir and ciclo-sporin (and possibly theophyllines). ↓s fx of rifampicin (rifampicin can also ↓fx of ketoconazole, as can phenytoin and clopidogrel), **W +**.

Dose: 200 mg od po *with food* (400 mg od in severe/resistant cases).

KLEAN-PREP see Bowel preparations.

Dose: up to 2 powder sachets the evening before and repeated on the morning of GI surgery or Ix.

LABETALOL

β-blocker with arteriolar vasodilatory properties ∴ also ⇒ ↓TPR.

Use: uncontrolled/severe HTN (inc during pregnancy[1] or post-MI[2] or with angina). *For advice on HTN Mx see p. 182.*

CI/Caution/SE/Interactions: as propranolol, plus can ⇒ 💀 severe/postural ↓BP 💀 and hepatotoxicity* (Ⓛ).

Monitor: LFTs* (if deteriorate stop drug).

Dose: initially 100 mg bd po (halve dose in elderly), ↑ing every fortnight if necessary to max of 600 mg qds po; if essential to ↓BP rapidly give 50 mg iv over ≥1 min repeating after 5 min if necessary (or can give 2 mg/min ivi), up to max total dose 200 mg; 20 mg/h ivi[1], doubling every 30 min to max of 160 mg/h; 15 mg/h ivi[2], ↑ing slowly to max of 120 mg/h. NB: consider ↓dose in RF.

LACRI-LUBE

Artificial tears for dry eyes.

SE: blurred vision ∴ usually used at bedtime (or if vision secondary consideration, e.g. Bell's palsy or blind eye).

Dose: 1 application prn.

LACTULOSE

Osmotic laxative[1]: bulking agent. Also ↓s growth of NH_4-producing bacteria[2].

Use: constipation[1], hepatic encephalopathy[2].

CI: GI obstruction, galactosaemia.

Caution: lactose intolerance.

SE: flatulence, distension, abdominal pains.

Dose: 15 ml od/bd[1] (↑dose according to response; NB: *can take 2 days to work*); 30–50 ml tds[2]. *Take with plenty of water.*

LAMISIL see Terbinafine.

▼ LAMOTRIGINE/LAMICTAL

Antiepileptic: ↓s release of excitatory amino acids (esp glutamate) via action on voltage-sensitive Na^+ channels.

Use: epilepsy (esp partial and 1° or 2° generalised tonic–clonic), Px depressive episode in bipolar disorder.

Caution: avoid abrupt withdrawal[†] (rebound seizure risk; taper off over ≥2 wks unless stopping due to serious skin reaction*), L/R/P/B/E.

SE: **cerebellar symptoms** (see p. 236), **skin reactions*** (often severe, e.g. SJS, TEN, lupus, esp in children, if on valproate, or high initial doses), **blood disorders**** (↓Hb, ↓WCC, ↓Pt), N&V. Rarely, ↓memory, sedation, Ψ disorders, sleep Δ, acne, pretibial ulcers, alopecia, worsening of seizures, poly-/an-uria, **hepatotoxicity**.

Monitor: U&Es, FBC, LFTs, clotting.

Warn: report rash* plus any 'flu-like symptoms, signs of infection/ ↓Hb or bruising**. Don't stop tablets suddenly[†]. Risk of suicidal ideation.

Interactions: fx are ↓d by OCP, phenytoin, carbamazepine, mefloquine, TCAs and SSRIs. fx ↑d by valproate.

Dose: 25–700 mg daily^{SPC/BNF}; ↑dose slowly to ↓risk of skin reactions* (also need to restart at low dose). **NB: ↓dose in LF.**

LANSOPRAZOLE/ZOTON

PPI. As omeprazole, but ↓interactions.
Dose: 15–30 mg od po (↓to 15 mg od for maintenance).

LARIAM see Mefloquine; antimalarial (Px and Rx).

LASIX see Furosemide; loop diuretic.

▼ LATANOPROST 0.01%/XALATAN

Topical PG analogue: ↑s uveoscleral outflow.
Use: ↑IOP in glaucoma and *ocular* HTN (1st line agent).
Caution: asthma (if severe), aphakia, pseudophakia, uveitis, macular oedema **P/B**.
SE: iris colour Δ* (can ⇒ permanent ↑brown pigmentation, esp if uniocular use), blurred vision, local reactions (e.g. conjunctival hyperaemia in up to 30% initially). Also darkening of periocular skin and ↑eyelash length (both reversible). Rarely cystoid macular oedema (if aphakia), uveitis, angina.
Warn: can Δ iris colour*.
Dose: 1 drop od.

LEFLUNOMIDE/ARAVA

DMARD; inhibits pyrimidine synthesis (also anti-inflammatory fx).
Use: active rheumatoid or psoriatic arthritis if standard DMARDs (e.g. methotrexate or sulfasalazine) CI or not tolerated.
CI: severe immunodeficiency, BM suppression, severe hypo-proteinaemia, serious infection, **L/R/P/B**.
Caution: blood disorders, recent hepato-/myelo-toxic drugs, TB (inc Hx of).
SE: BM toxicity, ↑risk of **infection/malignancy**, hepatotoxicity (potentially life-threatening in 1st 6 months), SJS, HTN.
Warn: teratogenic: must exclude pregnancy before starting Rx and use contraception during Rx (and until drug no longer active*).

Monitor: LFTs, FBC, BP.
Dose: specialist use only.

> Long $t_{1/2}$*: if serious SE discontinue treatment and needs prolonged washout period or active measures (e.g. cholestyramine 8 g tds or activated charcoal 50 g qds) to ↑elimination if wishing to conceive.

LEVOBUNOLOL

β-blocker eye drops: similar to timolol ⇒ ↓aqueous humour production. *Significant systemic absorption can occur.*
Use: chronic simple (wide-/open-angle) glaucoma.
CI/Caution/Interactions: as propranolol; interactions less likely.
SE: local reactions. Rarely anterior uveitis and anaphylaxis.
Can ⇒ systemic fx, esp bronchoconstriction/cardiac fx; see Propranolol.
Dose: 1 drop of 0.5% solution od/bd.

LEVODOPA (= L-DOPA)

Precursor of dopamine: needs concomitant peripheral dopa decarboxylase inhibitor such as benserazide (see Co-beneldopa) or carbidopa (see Co-careldopa) to limit SEs.
Use: Parkinsonism.
CI: glaucoma (closed-angle), taking MAO-A inhibitors*, melanoma†, **P/B**.
Caution: pulmonary/cardiovascular/Ψ disease, endocrine disorder, glaucoma (open angle), osteomalacia, Hx of PU or convulsions, ventricular arrhythmias, **L/R**.
SE: dyskinesias, abdominal upset, postural ↓BP/arrythmias, drowsiness, aggression, Ψ disorders (confusion, depression, suicide, hallucinations, psychosis, hypomania), seizures, dizziness, headache, flushing, sweating, peripheral neuropathy, taste Δs, rash/pruritus, can reactivate melanoma†, Δ LFTs, GI bleeding, blood disorders, dark body fluids (inc sweat).
Warn: can ⇒ daytime sleepiness (inc sudden-onset sleep) and ↓ability to drive/operate machinery.

Interactions: fx ↓d by neuroleptics, SEs ↑d by bupropion, **risk of ↑BP crisis with MAOIs*** (but can give with MAO-B inhibitors), risk of arrhythmias with halothane. **Dose:** 125–500 mg daily, *after food*, ↑ing according to response.

Abrupt withdrawal can ⇒ neuroleptic malignant-like syndrome.

LEVOMEPROMAZINE (= METHOTRIMEPRAZINE)

Phenothiazine antipsychotic; as chlorpromazine, but used in palliative care (see p. 189) as has good antiemetic[1] and sedative[2] fx, but little respiratory depression.
Use: refractory N&V[1] or restlessness/distress[2] in the terminally ill.
CI/Caution/SE/Interactions: as chlorpromazine, but ↑risk of postural ↓BP (esp in elderly: don't give if age >50 years and ambulant) and ↑risk of seizures (caution if epilepsy/brain tumour).
Dose: 6.25–25 mg po/sc/im/iv od/bd (can ↑to tds/qds), or 25–200 mg/ 24 h sc infusion. **Parenteral dose is half equivalent oral dose.** *NB: for N&V low doses may be effective and ⇒ ↓sedation. Doses >25 mg sc/ 24 hrs rarely needed except as major sedation.*
NB: ↓dose in RF and elderly.

LEVOTHYROXINE see Thyroxine.

LIBRIUM see Chlordiazepoxide; long-acting benzodiazepine.

LIDOCAINE (previously Lignocaine)
Class Ib antiarrhythmic (↓s conduction in Purkinje and ventricular muscle fibres), local anaesthetic (blocks axonal Na^+ channels).
Use: ventricular arrhythmias (esp post-MI), local anaesthesia.
CI: myocardial depression (if severe), SAN disorders, atrioventricular block (all grades), porphyria.
Caution: epilepsy, severe hypoxia/hypovolaemia/↓HR, **L/H/P/B/E.**
SE: dizziness, drowsiness, confusion, tinnitus, blurred vision, para-esthesia, GI upset, arrhythmias, ↓BP, ↓HR. Rarely respiratory depression, seizures, anaphylasis.
Monitor: ECG during iv administration.

L/R/H = Liver, Renal and Heart failure (full key see p. vii)

Interactions: ↑risk of arrhythmias with antipsychotics, dolasetron and quinu-/dalfo-pristin. ↑myocardial depression with other anti-arrhythmics and β-blockers. Levels ↑by propranolol, ataza-/lopi-navir and cimetidine. Prolongs action of suxamethonium.

Dose (*for ventricular arrhythmias*): 50–100 mg iv at rate of 25–30 mg/min followed immediately by ivi at 4 mg/min for 30 min then 2 mg/min for 2 h and 1 mg/min thereafter (↓dose further if drug needed for >24 h). NB: short $t_{1/2}$ ∴ if 15 min delay in setting up ivi, can give max 2 further doses of 50–100 mg iv ≥10 min apart. In emergencies, can often be found stocked in crash trolleys as Minijet syringes of 1% (10 mg/ml) or 2% (20 mg/ml) solutions.

☠ Local anaesthetic preparations must never be injected into veins or inflamed tissue, as can ⇒ systemic fx (esp arrhythmias) ☠.

LIGNOCAINE see Lidocaine.

LIOTHYRONINE (= L-TRI-IODOTHYRONINE) SODIUM

Synthetic T_3: quicker and more potent action than thyroxine (T_4).
Use: severe hypothyroidism (e.g. myxoedema coma*: see p. 257).
CI/Caution/SE/Interactions: see Thyroxine.
Dose: 5–20 microgram iv slowly. Repeat every 4–12 h as necessary; seek expert help. Also available po, but thyroxine (T_4) often preferred. NB: 20 microgram liothyronine = 100 microgram (levo)thyroxine.

Concurrent hydrocortisone iv is often also needed*; see p. 257.

LISINOPRIL

ACE-i; see Captopril.
Use: HTN[1] (*for advice on stepped HTN Mx see p. 182*), HF[2], Px of IHD post-MI[3], DM nephropathy[4].
CI/Caution/SE/Interactions: as Captopril.
Dose: initially 10 mg od[1] (2.5–5.0 mg if RF or used with diuretic) ↑ing if necessary to max 80 mg/day; initially 2.5–5 mg od[2,4] adjusted to response to usual maintenance of 5–20 mg/day. Doses post-MI[3] depend on BP[SPC/BNF].
NB: ↓dose in LF or RF.

LITHIUM

Mood stabiliser: modulates intracellular signalling; blocks neuronal Ca^{2+} channels and changes GABA pathways.

Use: mania Rx/Px, bipolar disorder Px. Rarely for recurrent depression Px and aggressive/self-mutilating behaviour Rx.

CI: ↓T_4 (if untreated), Addison's, SSS, cardiovascular disease, **P** (⇒ Ebstein's anomaly: esp in 1st trimester), **R/H/B**.

(NB: manufacturers don't agree on definitive list and all CI are **relative** – decisions should be made in clinical context and expert help sought if unsure.)

Caution: thyroid disease, MG, **E**.

SE: thirst, polyuria, GI upset (↑Wt, N&V&D), *fine tremor** (NB: in toxicity ⇒ *coarse* tremor), tardive dyskinesia, muscular weakness, acne, psoriasis exacerbation, ↑WCC, ↑Pt. Rarer but serious: ↓(or ↑) T_4 ± goitre (esp in females), renal impairment (diabetes insipidus, interstitial nephritis), arrhythmias. Very rarely can ⇒ neuroleptic malignant syndrome.

Monitor: serum levels *12 h post-dose*: keep at 0.6–1 mmol/l (>1.5 mmol/l may ⇒ toxicity, esp if elderly), U&Es, TFTs.

Warn: report symptoms of ↓T_4, avoid dehydration.

Interactions: toxicity (± levels) ↑d by **NSAIDs, diuretics*** (esp thiazides), SSRIs, ACE-i, ARBs, amiodarone, methyldopa, carbamazepine and haloperidol. Theophyllines, caffeine and antacids may ↓lithium levels.

Dose: see SPC/BNF: 2 *types* (salts) available with different doses ('carbonate' 200 mg = 'citrate' 509 mg) and bioavailabilities of particular *brands* vary ∴ *must specify salt and brand required*. For 'carbonate' starting dose usually 200 mg nocte, adjusting to plasma levels (maintenance usually 600 mg – 1 g nocte).

NB: ↓dose in LF.

Consider stopping 24 h before major surgery or ECT; restart once e'lytes return to normal. Discuss with anaesthetist ± psychiatrist.

L/R/H = **L**iver, **R**enal and **H**eart failure (full key see p. vii)

> **Lithium toxicity**
> *Features*: D&V, coarse tremor*, cerebellar signs (see p. 236), renal impairment/oliguria, ↓BP, ↑reflexes, convulsions, drowsiness ⇒ coma, arrhythmia. *Rx*: stop drug, control seizures, correct electrolytes (normally need saline ivi; high risk if ↓Na⁺: avoid low-salt diets and diuretics**). Consider haemodialysis if RF.

LOCOID see Hydrocortisone butyrate 0.1% (potent steroid) cream.

LOFEPRAMINE

2nd generation TCA.

Use: depression (see p. 197)

CI/Caution/SE/Warn/Monitor/Interactions: as amitriptyline but also **R** (if severe). Also ⇒ ↓sedation (sometimes alerting – don't give nocte if occurs) and ↓anticholinergic and cardiac SEs ∴ ↓*danger in* OD.

Dose: 140–210 mg daily in divided (bd/tds) doses.

LOPERAMIDE/IMODIUM

Antimotility agent: synthetic opioid analogue; binds to receptors in GI muscle ⇒ ↓peristalsis, ↑transit time, ↑H₂O/electrolyte resorption, ↓gut secretions, ↑sphincter tone. Extensive 1st-pass metabolism ⇒ minimal systemic opioid fx.

Use: diarrhoea.

CI: constipation, ileus, megacolon, bacterial enterocolitis 2° to invasive organisms (e.g. salmonella, *Shigella*, *Campylobacter*), abdominal distension, active UC/AAC, pseudomembranous colitis.

Caution: in young (can ⇒ fluid + electrolyte depletion), **L/P**.

SE: constipation, abdominal cramps, bloating, dizziness, drowsiness, fatigue. Rarely hypersensitivity (esp skin reactions), paralytic ileus.

Dose: initially 4 mg, then 2 mg after each loose stool (max 16 mg/day for 5 days). *NB: can mask serious GI conditions.*

LORATADINE

Non-sedating antihistamine: see Cetirizine.

Dose: 10 mg od. Non-proprietary or as Clarityn.

LORAZEPAM

Benzodiazepine, short-acting (see p. 229).
Use: sedation[1] (esp acute behavioural disturbance/Ψ disorders, e.g. acute psychosis), status epilepticus[2].
CI/Caution/SE/Interactions: see Diazepam.
Dose: 0.5–2 mg po/im/iv prn (bottom of this range if elderly/ respiratory disease/naive to benzodiazepines; top of range if young/ recent exposure to benzodiazepines; max 4 mg/day)[1]; 0.1 mg/kg ivi at 2 mg/min (max 4 mg repeated once after 10 mins if necessary)[2]. **NB:** ↓dose in RF.

> ☠ Beware respiratory depression: have O_2 (± resuscitation trolley) at hand, esp if respiratory disease or giving high doses im/iv ☠.

▼ LOSARTAN/COZAAR

Angiotensin II receptor antagonist: specifically blocks renin–angiotensin system ∴ does not inhibit bradykinin and ⇒ dry cough.
Use: HTN (*for advice on stepped HTN Mx see p. 182*), Px of type 2 DM nephropathy (if ACE-i not tolerated*).
CI: P/B.
Caution: RAS, HOCM, mitral/aortic stenosis, if taking drugs that ↑K^+**, **L/R/E.**
SE/Interactions: as captopril, but ↓dry cough (major reason for ACE-i intolerance*). As with ACE-i, can ⇒ ↑K^+(esp if taking ↑K^+ sparing diuretics/salt substitutes or if RF).
Dose: initially 25–50 mg od (↑ing to max 100 mg od). **NB:** ↓dose in LF or RF.

> ☠ **Beware if on other drugs that ↑K^+, e.g. amiloride, spironolactone, triamterene, ACE-i and ciclosporin. Don't give with oral K^+ supplements (inc dietary salt substitutes) ☠.

LOSEC see Omeprazole; PPI (ulcer-healing drug).

LUGOL'S SOLUTION

Oral I_2 solution (containing iodine and K^+ iodide).
Use: ↑T_4 if severe ('thyroid storm' see p. 256) or pre-operatively.

CI: B.
Caution: not for long-term Rx, **P**.
SE: hypersensitivity.
Dose: 0.1–0.3 ml tds (of solution containing 130 mg iodine/ml).

LYMECYCLINE

Tetracycline, broad-spectrum antibiotic (see Tetracycline).
Use: acne vulgaris, rosacea.
CI/Caution/SE/Interactions: as tetracycline.
Dose: 408 mg od for ≥8 wks (can ↑to bd for other indications).

MADOPAR see Co-beneldopa; L-dopa for Parkinson's.

MAGNESIUM SULPHATE (iv)

Mg^{2+} replacement.
Use: life-threatening asthma[1] (unlicensed indication), serious arrhythmias[2] (esp if torsades or if ↓K^+; often caused by ↓Mg^{2+}), MI[3] (equivocal evidence of ↓mortality), eclampsia/pre-eclampsia[4] (↓s seizures), symptomatic ↓Mg^{2+}[5] (mostly 2° to GI loss).
Caution: monitor BP, respiratory rate and urine output, **L/R**.
SE: flushing, ↓BP, GI upset, thirst, ↓reflexes, weakness, confusion/drowsiness. Rarely arrhythmias, respiratory depression, coma.
Interactions: ↑risk of ↓BP with Ca^{2+} channel blockers.
Dose: 4–8 mmol ivi over 20 min[1]; 8 mmol iv over 10–15 min[2] (repeating once if required); 8 mmol ivi over 20 min then ivi of 65–72 mmol over 24 h[3]; 4 mg ivi over 5–10 min then ivi at 1 mg/h until 24 hr after the last seizure[4]; up to 160 mmol ivi/im according to need[5] (over up to 5 days). For iv injection, use concentrations of ≤20%; if using 50% solution dilute 1 part with ≥1.5 parts water for injection.

MANNITOL

Osmotic diuretic.
Use: cerebral oedema[1] (and glaucoma).
CI: pulmonary oedema, **H**.
SE: GI upset, fever/chills, oedema. Rarely seizures, HF.

Dose: 0.25–2 g/kg as rapid ivi over 30–60 min[1].

MAXOLON see Metoclopramide; antiemetic (DA antagonist).

MEBEVERINE

Antispasmodic: direct action on GI muscle.
Use: GI smooth-muscle cramps (esp IBS, diverticulitis).
CI: ileus (paralytic).
Caution: porphyria, **P**.
SE: hypersensitivity/skin reactions.
Dose: 135–150 mg tds (20 min before food) or 200 mg bd of SR preparation (Colofac MR).

MEFENAMIC ACID/PONSTAN

Mild NSAID; non-selective COX inhibitor.
Use: musculoskeletal pain, dysmenorrhoea, menorrhagia.
CI/Caution/SE/Interactions: as ibuprofen, but also CI if IBD, caution if epilepsy or acute porphyria. Can ⇒ severe diarrhoea, skin reactions, stomatitis, paraesthesia, fatigue, haemolytic/aplastic ↓Hb, ↓Pt. No known interaction with baclofen or triazoles. Mild **W** +.
Dose: 500 mg tds.

MEFLOQUINE/LARIAM

Antimalarial; kills asexual forms of *Plasmodium*.
Use: malaria Px[1] (in areas of chloroquine-resistant falciparum spp) and rarely as Rx *if not taking the drug as Px*.
CI: hypersensitivity *to mefloquine or quinine*, Hx of neuro-Ψ disorders (inc depression, convulsions).
Caution: epilepsy, cardiac conduction disorders, **L/P/B**.
SE: GI upset, **neuro-Ψ reactions** (dizziness, ↓balance, headache, convulsions, sleep disorders, neuropathies, tremor, anxiety, depression, psychosis, hallucinations, panic attacks, agitation). Also cardiac fx (AV block, other conduction disorders, ↑ or ↓HR, ↑or ↓BP), hypersensitivity reactions.
Warn: can ↓driving/other skilled tasks and ⇒ neuro-Ψ reactions.

Interactions: ↑risk of seizures with quinine, chloroquine and hydroxychloroquine. ↓s fx of anticonvulsants (esp valproate and carbamazepine). ↑risk of arrhythmias with amiodarone, quinidine, moxifloxacin and pimozide. Avoid artemether/lumefantrine.
Dose: 250 mg once-wkly[1] (↓dose if Wt <45 kg)$^{SPC/BNF}$.

Need to start Px 2 1/2 wks before entering endemic area (to identify neuro-Ψ reactions; 75% of reactions occur by 3rd dose) and continue for 4 wks after leaving endemic area.

MEROPENEM

Carbapenem broad-spectrum antibiotic (β-lactam, but non-penicillin/non-cephalosporin).
Use: severe Gram +ve and −ve aerobic and anaerobic infections. Hospital acquired septicaemia.
Caution: β-lactam sensitivity (avoid if immediate hypersensitivity reaction) L/R/P/B.
SE: GI upset (N&V&D – inc AAC), ΔLFTs, headache, blood/skin disorders. Rarely seizures, SJS/TENS.
Monitor: LFTs.
Dose: 500 mg tds iv/ivi (↑to 1 g tds if severe infection or 2 g tds if meningitis or exacerbation of lower RTI in CF).
NB: ↑interval ± ↓dose if RF$^{SPC/BNF}$.

MESALAZINE

'New' aminosalicylate: as sulfasalazine, but with ↓sulphonamide SEs.
Use: UC (Rx/maintenance of remission).
CI: *hypersensitivity to any salicylates*, coagulopathies, **R** (caution only if mild), **L** (caution only if not severe).
Caution: P/B/E.
SE: GI upset, blood disorders, hypersensitivity (inc lupus), RF.
Warn: report unexplained bleeding, bruising, fever, sore throat or malaise.
Monitor: U&E, FBC (stop drug if blood disorder suspected).
Interactions: fx ↓by lactulose. NSAIDs and azathioprine may ↑nephrotoxicity.

Dose: as Asacol (or Ipocol, Mezavant, Mesren, Pentasa and Salofalk). Preparations not interchangeable as delivery characteristics may vary.

MESNA

Binds to metabolite (acrolein) of thiol-containing chemotherapy agents (cyclophosphamide, ifosfamide), which are toxic to urothelium and can ⇒ severe haemorrhagic cystitis. Give as Px before chemotherapy; see BNF for details.

METFORMIN

Oral antidiabetic (biguanide): ⇒ ↑insulin sensitivity w/o affecting levels (⇒ ↓gluconeogenesis and ↓GI absorption of glucose and ↑peripheral use of glucose). Only active in presence of endogenous insulin (i.e. functional islet cells).

Use: type 2 DM: usually 1st-line if diet control unsuccessful (esp if obese, as ⇒ less ↑Wt than sulphonylureas). Also used in PCOS (unlicensed; specialist use).

CI: DKA, ↑risk of lactic acidosis (e.g. RF, severe dehydration/ infection/peripheral vascular disease, shock, major trauma, respiratory failure, alcohol dependence, **recent MI*, general anaesthetic** or iodine-containing radiology contrast media***), **L/R/P/B**.

SE: GI upset (esp initially or if ↑doses), taste disturbance. Rarely ↓vit B$_{12}$ absorption, lactic acidosis[†] (stop drug).

Dose: Standard release tablets – initially 500 mg mane, ↑ing as required to max 2 g/day in divided doses. Modified release tablets – initially 500 mg daily, ↑ing as required to max 2 g daily in 1. *Take with meals.* NB: ↓dose in mild RF, avoid in severe RF.

> 🐛 *Both often coexist in coronary angiography: stop drug on day of procedure (giving insulin if necessary; see p. 203) and restart 48 h later, having checked that renal function has not deteriorated. Stop on day of surgery ahead of general anaesthetic** and restart when renal function normal 🐛.

METHADONE

Opioid agonist: ↓euphoria and long $t_{1/2}$ (⇒ ↓withdrawal symptoms) compared with other opioids.

Use: opioid dependence as aid to withdrawal.

CI/Caution/SE/Interactions: as morphine but levels not ↑by ritonavir, but are by voriconazole and cimetidine and ↑risk of ventricular arrhythmias with atomoxetine and amisulpride. Can ↑QTc (caution if family history of sudden death).

Dose: *individual requirements vary widely according to level of previous abuse*: sensible starting dose is 10–20 mg/day po, ↑ing by 10–20 mg every day until no signs or symptoms of withdrawal – which usually stop at 60–120 mg/day. Then aim to wean off gradually. Available as non-proprietary solutions (1 mg/ml) or as Methadose (10 mg/ml or 20 mg/ml). Can give sc/im[SPC/BNF]. **NB:** ↓dose if LF, RF or elderly.

☠ Don't confuse solutions of different strengths ☠.

METHIONINE

Sulphur-containing amino acid: binds toxic metabolites of paracetamol.

Use: paracetamol OD *<12 h post-ingestion* (ineffective after this) and not vomiting, mostly when acetylcysteine ivi cannot be given (e.g. outside hospital).

CI: metabolic acidosis.

Caution: schizophrenia (can worsen), L.

SE: N&V, irritability, drowsiness.

Interactions: can ↓fx of L-dopa.

Dose: 2.5 g po 4-hrly (for *4 doses only: total dose = 10 g*).

METHOTREXATE

Immunosuppressant, antimetabolite: dihydrofolate reductase inhibitor (↓s nucleic acid synthesis).

Use: rheumatoid arthritis[1] (1st-line DMARD) and other inflammatory joint and muscle disorders, **psoriasis** (if severe/resistant), **Ca** (ALL, non-Hodgkin's lymphoma, choriocarcinoma, various solid tumours), rarely in Crohn's disease.

CI: severe blood disorders, active infections, immunodeficiency, **R/L** (if either significant, otherwise caution), **P** (females and *males* must avoid conception for ≥ 3 months after stopping treatment), **B**.

Caution: effusions (esp ascites and pleural effusions: drain before starting treatment as risk of ↑toxicity), ↑ rheumatoid nodules, blood disorders, UC, PU, ↓immunity, porphyria, **E**.

SE: mucositis/GI upset, myelosuppression, skin reactions. Rarely **pulmonary fibrosis/pneumonitis** (esp in RA), liver toxicity/ hepatic fibrosis (esp in psoriatics), neurotoxicity (inc necrotising demyelinating leukoencephalopathy), seizures, RF (esp tubular necrosis).

Monitor: U&Es, FBC, LFTs $\pm$ procollagen 3 protein (to monitor for hepatic fibrosis).

Interactions: NSAIDs (e.g. concomitant use in RA), **trimethoprim, co-trimoxazole,** corticosteroids (e.g concomitant use in RA), probenecid, nitrous oxide, pyrimethamine, clozapine, cisplatin, acitretin, ciclosporin all ⇒ ↑toxicity $\pm$ levels.

Warn: avoid over-the-counter NSAIDs*, report any clinical features of infection (esp sore throat).

Dose: Oral: start 7.5 mg once weekly (max oral weekly dose 20 mg)[1]. For other indications and routes see BNF/SPC. NB: ↓dose in RF. *Usually needs concomitant folic acid (range 5 mg once/wk–5 days/wk (omitted day of and day after, methotrexate)).*

☠NB: dose is only once a week: potentially fatal if given daily☠.

METHOTRIMEPRAZINE see Levomepromazine; DA antagonist.

METHYLDOPA

Centrally acting α_2 agonist.

Use: HTN; esp pregnancy-induced and 1° HTN during pregnancy. *For advice on HTN Mx see p. 182.*

CI: depression, phaeo, porphyria, **L** (if active liver disease).

Caution: Hx of depression/**L**, **R**.

SE: (minimal if dose <1 g/day) dry mouth, sedation, dizziness, weakness, headache, GI upset, postural ↓BP, ↓HR. Rarely **blood disorders**, **hepatotoxicity**, pancreatitis, Ψ disorders, Parkinsonism, lupus-like syndrome, false +ve direct Coombs' test.

Monitor: FBC, LFTs.

Interactions: ↑s neurotoxicity of lithium. Hypotensive fx ↑d by antidepressants, anaesthetics and salbutamol ivi. ☠ **Avoid with, or within 2 wks of, MAOIs** ☠.

Dose: initially 250 mg bd/tds (125 mg bd in elderly), ↑ing gradually at intervals ≥2 days (max 2 g/day in elderly) to max of 3 g/day. **NB:** ↓dose in RF.

METHYLPREDNISOLONE

Glucocorticoid (mild mineralocorticoid activity).

Use: acute flares of inflammatory diseases[1] (esp rheumatoid arthritis, MS), cerebral oedema, Rx of graft rejection.

CI/Caution/SE/Interactions: see Steroids section (p. 225).

Dose: acutely, 250 mg–1 g ivi od[1] (normally for 3 days). Also available po and as im depot.

METOCLOPRAMIDE/MAXOLON

Antiemetic: D_2 antagonist: acts on central chemoreceptor trigger zone and directly stimulates GI tract (⇒ ↑motility).

Use: N&V, esp GI (gastroduodenal, biliary, hepatic) or opiate-/chemotherapy-induced.

CI: GI obstruction/perforation/haemorrhage (inc 3–4 days post-GI surgery), phaeo, **B**.

Caution: epilepsy, porphyria, L/R/P/E.

SE: extrapyramidal fx (see p. 236 – esp in elderly and young females: reversible if drug stopped w/in 24 h or with procyclidine), **drowsiness**, restlessness, GI upset, behavioural/mood Δs, ↑prolactin. Rarely skin reactions, neuroleptic malignant syndrome.

Interactions: ↑s fx of NSAIDs and ciclosporin levels. ↑s risk of extrapyramidal fx of antipsychotics, SSRIs and TCAs.

Dose: 10 mg tds po/sc/im/iv. **NB:** ↓dose in RF, LF.

METOLAZONE

Potent thiazide-like diuretic: as bendroflumethiazide, plus has additive diuretic fx with loop diuretics.

Use: oedema[1], HTN[2] (*for advice on stepped HTN Mx see p. 182*).
CI/Caution/SE/Interactions: see Bendroflumethiazide.
Monitor: e'lytes (esp Na^+/K^+) closely.
Dose: 5–10 mg od po (mane), ↑ing if needed to max of 80 mg/day (rarely >20 mg/day[1]); initially 5 mg od, then on alternate days for maintenance[2].

METOPROLOL

β-Blocker, cardioselective ($\beta_1 > \beta_2$), short-acting.
Use: HTN[1] (*for advice on stepped HTN Mx see p. 182*), angina[2], arrhythmias[3], migraine Px[4], ↑T_4 (adjunct)[5].
CI/Caution/SE/Interactions: see Propranolol.
Dose: 50–100 mg bd po[1,4]; 50–100 mg bd/tds po[2,3]; 50 mg qds po[5]. Can give 2–5 mg iv[SPC/BNF] repeating to max 10–15 mg. See p. 240 for use in AMI/ACS. **NB:** ↓dose in LF.

METRONIDAZOLE/FLAGYL

Antibiotic, 'cidal': binds DNA of anaerobic (and microaerophilic) bacteria/protozoa.
Use: **anaerobic and protozoal infections**, abdominal sepsis (esp *Bacteroides*), aspiration pneumonia, *C. difficile* (AAC), *H. pylori* eradication (see p. 177), *Giardia/Entamoeba* infections, Px during GI surgery. Also dental/gynaecological infections, bacterial vaginosis (*Gardnerella*), PID.
Caution: **avoid with alcohol**: drug metabolised to acetaldehyde and other toxins ⇒ flushing, abdominal pain, ↓BP ('disulfiram-like' reaction), acute porphyria, **L/P/B**.
SE: GI upset (esp N&V), taste disturbed, skin reactions. Rarely, drowsiness, headache, dizziness, dark urine, hepatotoxicity, blood disorders, myalgia, arthralgia, seizures (transient), ataxia, **peripheral neuropathy** (if prolonged Rx).
Interactions: can ↑busulfan, lithium and phenytoin levels, **W** + .

Dose: 500 mg tds ivi/400 mg tds po for severe infections. Lower doses can be given po or higher doses pr (1 g bd/tds) according to indication[SPC/BNF]. **NB:** ↓dose in LF.

MICONAZOLE

Imidazole antifungal (topical) but *systemic absorption can occur*.

Use: oral fungal infections (give po), cutaneous fungal infections (give topically).

CI: L. Oral gel – in infants: impaired swallowing reflex, and up to 5–6 months if born pre-term.

Caution: acute porphyria, **P/B**.

SE: GI upset. Rarely hypersensitivity, hepatotoxicity.

Interactions: as ketoconazole, but less commonly significant. **W** + .

Dose: **po:** oral gel (Daktarin) 5–10 ml qds (after food); 2.5 mg bd (4 months–2 yrs), 5 mg bd (2–6 yrs), 5 mg qds (6 yrs +) or buccal tablets (▼ Loramyc) 50 mg od mane. **top:** apply 1–2 times/day.

MIDAZOLAM

Benzodiazepine, very short-acting (see p. 229).

Use: sedation for stressful/painful procedures[1] (esp if amnesia desirable) and for agitation/distress in palliative care[2].

CI/Caution/SE/Warn/Interactions: see Diazepam.

Dose: 1.0–7.5 mg iv[1]; initially 2 mg (0.5–1 mg if elderly) over 60 sec, then titrate up slowly until desired sedation achieved using 0.5–1.0-mg boluses over 30 sec (can also give im[SPC/BNF]); 2.5–5 mg sc prn[2] (or via sc pump; see p. 189). Also available as buccal liquid (10 mg/ml, special preparation) – unlicensed use. **NB:** ↓dose in RF or elderly.

☠ Beware respiratory depression: have flumazenil and O_2 (± resuscitation trolley) at hand, esp if respiratory disease or giving high doses im/iv☠.

MINOCYCLINE

Tetracycline antibiotic: inhibits ribosomal (30S subunit) protein synthesis; broadest spectrum of tetracyclines.

Use: acne[1], rosacea.

CI/Caution/SE/Interactions: as tetracycline, but ↓bacterial resistance, although ↑risk of SLE and irreversible skin/body fluid discoloration. Can also use (with caution) in RF. Check hepatic toxicity every 3 months – discontinue if develops.

Dose: 100 mg od po[1] (can ↑to bd for other indications). Use for ≥3 months in acne.

MINOXIDIL

Peripheral vasodilator (arterioles >> veins): also ⇒ ↑CO, ↑HR, fluid retention ∴ *always needs concurrent β-blocker and diuretic.*
Use: HTN (if severe/Rx-resistant); *for HTN Mx advice see p. 182.*
CI: phaeo.
Caution: IHD, acute porphyria, R/P/B.
SE: hypertrichosis, coarsening of facial features (reversible, but makes it less suitable for women), ↑Wt, peripheral oedema, pericardial effusions, angina (dt ↑HR). Rarely, GI upset, gynaecomastia/breast tenderness, renal impairment, skin reactions.
Dose: initially 2.5–5 mg/day in 1 or 2 divided doses, ↑ing by 5–10 mg at an interval of at least 3 days if needed up to usual max of 50 mg/day. NB: ↓**dose in elderly and dialysis patients.** Also used topically for male-pattern baldness.

MIRTAZAPINE/ZISPIN

Antidepressant: **N**oradrenaline **A**nd **S**pecific **S**erotonin **A**gonist (NASSA); specifically stimulates $5HT_1$ receptors (antagonises $5HT_{2C}/5HT_3$), antagonises central presynaptic α_2 receptors.
Use: depression, esp in elderly* or if insomnia[†] see p. 197.
CI/Caution/SE: as fluoxetine, but ⇒ ↓**sexual dysfunction**/GI upset, ↑**sedation**[†] (esp during titration) and ↑**appetite/Wt** (can be beneficial in elderly*). Rarely, blood disorders (inc agranulocytosis**), Δ LFTs, convulsions, myoclonus, oedema.
Warn: of initial sedation, to not stop suddenly (risk of withdrawal; see p. 235) and to report signs of infection** (esp sore throat, fever): stop drug and check FBC if concerned.

L/R/H = Liver, Renal and Heart failure (full key see p. vii)

Interactions: avoid with other sedatives (inc alcohol), artemether/lumefantrine. ☠ **Never give with, or ≤2 wks after, MAOIs** ☠.
Dose: initially 15 mg nocte ↑ing to 30 mg after 1–2 wks (max 45 mg/day). *Note lower doses more sedating than higher doses.*

MISOPROSTOL

Synthetic PGE$_1$ analogue: ↓s gastric acid secretion.
Use: Px/Rx of PU (esp NSAID-induced). Unlicensed uses: po or topically to cervix for induction of labour, to induce medical abortion and to ripen cervix for surgical abortion; also pr in postpartum haemorrhage.
CI: ☠ **pregnancy** ☠ (actual or planned; only give to women of childbearing age if high risk of PU and contraceptives prescribed), **P/B**.
Caution: cardiovascular/cerebrovascular disease (can ⇒ ↓BP), IBD.
SE: diarrhoea. Rarely, other GI upset, rash, light-headedness, menstrual Δs, vaginal bleeding.
Warn: women of child-bearing age of risks to pregnancy and need for adequate contraception when taking.
Dose: most often used with diclofenac as Arthrotec. Also available with naproxen as Napratec. Both these preparations contain 200 microgram misoprostol per tablet, i.e. total daily dose < the ideal 800 microgram.

MMF see Mycophenolate mofetil; immunosuppressant.

MOMETASONE (FUROATE) CREAM OR OINTMENT/ ELOCON

Potent topical corticosteroid.
Use: inflammatory skin conditions, esp eczema.
CI: untreated infection, rosacea, acne.
SE: skin atrophy, worsening of infections, acne.
Dose: apply thinly od top (use 'ointment' in dry skin conditions).

MONTELUKAST/SINGULAIR

Leukotriene receptor antagonist: ↓s Ag-induced bronchoconstriction.

Use: *non-acute* asthma (see BTS guidelines, p. 186), esp if large exercise-induced component or associated seasonal allergic rhinitis.

Caution: acute asthma, Churg–Strauss syndrome **P/B**.

SE: headache, GI upset, myalgia, dry mouth/thirst. Rarely **Churg–Strauss syndrome**: asthma ($\pm$ rhin-/sinus-itis) with systemic vasculitis and ↑EØ*.

Monitor: FBC* and for development of vasculitic (purpuric/non-blanching) rash, peripheral neuropathy, ↑respiratory/cardiac symptoms: all signs of possible Churg–Strauss syndrome.

Dose: 10 mg nocte (↓doses if <15 years old[SPC/BNF]).

MORPHGESIC SR Morphine (sulphate) SR (10, 30, 60 or 100 mg). Given bd. NB: ↓dose if LF, RF or elderly.

MORPHINE (SULPHATE)

Opiate analgesic.

Use: severe pain (inc post-op), AMI and acute LVF.

CI: acute respiratory depression, acute severe obstructive airways disease, ↑risk of paralytic ileus, delayed gastric emptying, biliary colic, acute alcoholism, ↑ICP/head injury (respiratory depression $\Rightarrow CO_2$ retention and cerebral vasodilation $\Rightarrow$ ↑ICP), phaeo. **H** (if 2° to chronic lung disease).

Caution: ↓respiratory reserve, obstructive airways disease, ↓BP/shock, acute abdomen, biliary tract disorders (NB: biliary colic is CI), pancreatitis, bowel obstruction, IBD, ↑prostate/urethral stricture, arrhythmias, ↓T$_4$, adrenocorticoid insufficiency, MG, **L** (can $\Rightarrow$ coma), **R/P/B/E**.

SE: N&V (and other GI disturbance) constipation* (can $\Rightarrow$ ileus), respiratory depression, ↓BP (inc orthostatic. NB: rarely $\Rightarrow$ ↑BP), ↓/↑HR, pulmonary oedema, oedema, bronchospasm, ↓cough reflex, sedation, urinary retention, RF, biliary tract spasm, ↑pancreatitis, ΔLFTs, hypothermia, muscle rigidity/fasciculation/myoclonus, ↑ICP, dry mouth, vertigo, syncope, headache, miosis, sensory disturbance, pruritis, anorexia, allodynia, mood Δ(↑ or ↓), delirium, hallucinations, restlessness, seizures (at ↑doses), rhabdomyolysis, amenorrhoea, ↓libido, **dependence**. Rarely, skin reactions.

Interactions: ☠ MAOIs (don't give within 2 wks of) ☠. Levels ↓by ritonavir. ↓s levels of ciprofloxacin. ↑sedative fx with antihistamines, baclofen, alcohol (also ⇒ ↓BP), TCAs, antipsychotics (also ↓BP), anxiolytics/hypnotics, barbiturates and moclobemide (also ⇒ ↑CNS and ↑/↓BP). ↑s fx of sodium oxybate, gabapentin.

Dose: Acute pain: 5–20 mg sc/im 4-hrly; 2.5–15 mg iv up to 4-hrly (2 mg/min). NB: iv doses are generally 1/4–1/2 im doses. **AMI:** 5–10 mg iv (1–2 mg/min), repeated if necessary. **Acute LVF:** 5–10 mg iv (2 mg/min). **Chronic pain:** use po as Oramorph solution or as MST Continus, Morphgesic, MXL, Sevredol or Zomorph tablets – see p. 189; dose adjustment may be required when switching brands. Also available pr as suppositories of 10, 15, 20 and 30 mg giving 15–30 mg up to 4-hrly. *Unless short-term Rx, always consider laxative Px**. Can ↑doses and frequency with expert supervision. Always adjust dose to response. **NB: ↓dose if LF, RF or elderly.**

☠ If ↓BMI or elderly, titrate dose up slowly, monitor O₂ sats and have naloxone ± resuscitation trolley at hand ☠.

MST CONTINUS Oral morphine (sulphate), equivalent in efficacy to Oramorph but SR: dose every 12 hrs. Need to specify if *tablets* (5, 10, 15, 30, 60, 100 or 200 mg) or *suspension* (sachets of 20, 30, 60, 100 or 200 mg to be mixed with water). See also Palliative Care (p. 189).

MUPIROCIN/BACTROBAN

Topical antibiotic for bacterial infections (esp eradication of nasal MRSA carriage); available as nasal ointment, applied bd/tds.

Local MRSA eradication protocols often exist; if not, then a sensible regimen is to give for 5 days and then swab 2 days later, repeating regimen if culture still positive.

MXL CAPSULES Morphine (sulphate) capsules (30, 60, 90, 120, 150 or 200 mg), equivalent in efficacy to Oramorph but SR: dose od. See also Palliative Care (p. 189). NB: ↓dose if LF, RF or elderly.

MYCOPHENOLATE MOFETIL (MMF)

Immunosuppressant: $\downarrow$s B-/T-cell lymphocytes (and $\downarrow$s Ab production by B-cells).

Use: transplant rejection Px, autoimmune diseases, vasculitis.

CI: P/B

Caution: active serious GI diseases[†], **E**.

Monitor: FBC and LFTs (2-wkly for 2 months, then monthly for 1st year).

Warn: patient to report unexplained bruises/bleeding/signs of infection. Avoid strong sunlight*.

SE: GI upset, blood disorders (esp $\downarrow$NØ, $\downarrow$Pt), weakness, tremor, headache, $\uparrow$cholesterol, $\uparrow$or $\downarrow$K$^+$. Rarely GI ulceration/bleeding/perforation[†], hepatotoxicity, skin neoplasms*.

Interactions: $\uparrow$risk of agranulocytosis with clozapine. Levels $\downarrow$by rifampicin.

Dose: Specialist use only[SPC/BNF].

N-ACETYLCYSTEINE see Acetylcysteine; paracetamol antidote.

NALOXONE

Opioid receptor antagonist for opiate reversal if OD or over-Rx.

Caution: cardiovascular disease, if taking cardiotoxic drugs, physical dependence on opioids, **H**.

Dose: 0.4–2 mg iv (or sc/im), much larger doses may be needed for certain opioids (e.g. tramadol), repeating after 2 min if no response (or $\uparrow$ing if severe poisoning). NB: *Short-acting*: may need repeating every 2–3 min (to total 10 mg) then review and consider ivi (10 mg made up to 50 ml with 5% dextrose; useful start rate is 60% of initial dose over 1 h, then adjusted to response).

NALTREXONE

Opioid antagonist: $\downarrow$s euphoria of opioids if dependence and $\downarrow$s craving and relapse rate in alcoholic withdrawal (opioids thought to mediate alcohol addiction; not licensed for this in UK yet).

Use: Opioid and alcohol withdrawal; start >1 wk after stopping*.
CI: if still taking opioids (can precipitate withdrawal*), **L** (inc acute hepatitis).
Caution: R/P/B.
SE: GI upset, **hepatoxicity**, sleep and Ψ disorders.
Monitor: LFTs.
Warn: patient that trying to overcome opiate blockade OD can ⇒ acute intoxication.
Dose: initial dose 25 mg od po, thereafter 50 mg od (or 350 mg per week split into 2 × 100 mg and 1 × 150 mg doses); specialist use only.

NB: also ↓s fx of opioid analgesics.

NAPROXEN

Moderate-strength NSAID; non-selective COX inhibitor.
Use: rheumatic disease[1]; acute musculoskeletal pain and dysmenorrhoea[2]; acute gout[3].
CI/Caution/SE/Interactions: as ibuprofen, but somewhat ↑SEs, notably, ↑risk PU/GI bleeds. Lowest thrombotic risk of any NSAID. Probenecid ⇒ ↑serum levels. No known interaction with baclofen or triazoles. Mild **W** + .
Dose: 500 mg–1 g daily in 1–2 divided doses[1]; 500 mg initially then 250 mg 6–8-hrly (max 1.25 g/day)[2]; 750 mg initially then 250 mg 8-hrly[3]. Also available with misoprostol as Px against PU (as Napratec). NB: Avoid or ↓dose in RF & consider **gastroprotective Rx**.

NARATRIPTAN/NARAMIG

5HT$_{1B/1D}$ agonist for acute migraine.
CI/Caution/SE/Interactions: see Sumatriptan.
Dose: 2.5 mg po (can repeat after ≥4 h if responded then recurs). Max 5 mg/24 h (2.5 mg if LF or RF, avoid if severe).

NARCAN see Naloxone; opiate antidote.

NICORANDIL

K^+-channel activator ($\Rightarrow$ arterial dilation $\Rightarrow$ $\downarrow$afterload) with nitrate component ($\Rightarrow$ venous dilation $\Rightarrow$ $\downarrow$preload).

Use: angina Px/Rx (unresponsive to other Rx).

CI: $\downarrow$BP (esp cardiogenic shock), LVF with $\downarrow$filling pressures, **B**.

Caution: hypovolaemia, acute pulmonary oedema, ACS with LVF and $\downarrow$filling pressures, **P**.

SE: headache (often only initially*), **flushing**, dizziness, weakness, N&V, $\downarrow$BP, $\uparrow$HR (dose-dependent). Rarely GI/perianal ulcers (consider stopping drug), myalgia, angioedema, hepatotoxicity.

Interactions: ☠ risk of $\downarrow\downarrow$BP with silden-/tadal-/varden-afil ☠.

Dose: 5–30 mg bd (start low, esp if susceptible to headaches*).

NICOTINIC ACID/NIASPAN

Water-soluble B-complex vitamin; $\downarrow$s synthesis of cholesterol/TGs and $\uparrow$s HDL-cholesterol.

Use: dyslipidaemia ($\uparrow$cholesterol, $\uparrow$TG, $\downarrow$HDL-cholesterol) *added to statin or if statin not tolerated*.

CI: active bleeding, active PU disease. **L**(if severe)/**B**.

Caution: ACS, gout, history of PU, $\uparrow$alcohol intake, DM. **R/P**.

SE: GI upset, dyspepsia, flushing, itch, rash, headache $\uparrow$HR, $\downarrow$BP, syncope, SOB, oedema, $\uparrow$uric acid, $\uparrow$INR, $\downarrow$Pt, $\downarrow$phosphate, DM, muscle disorders. Rarely rhabdomyolysis, anorexia.

Warn: avoid alcohol or hot drink around time of tablet ($\uparrow$flushing and itch); false +ve urine G result. Flushing prostaglandin mediated; can be avoided if darrow; initial dose taken with meals, or if taking aspirin give 30 mins before nicotinic acid.

Monitor: BG, CK (if $\uparrow$risk myopathy) and LFTs (if mild-moderate LF).

Interactions: $\uparrow$risk of myopathy with statins.

Dose: 375 mg (MR tablets) od nocte after low fat snack; $\uparrow$dose weekly for 4 wks then monthly if needed. Maintenance dose 1–2 g od nocte.

NIFEDIPINE

Ca^{2+} channel blocker (dihydropyridine): dilates smooth muscle, esp arteries (inc coronaries). Reflex sympathetic drive $\Rightarrow$ ↑HR and ↑contractility ∴ $\Rightarrow$ ↓HF cf other Ca^{2+} channel blockers (e.g. verapamil, and to a lesser degree diltiazem), which $\Rightarrow$ ↓HR + ↓contractility. Also diuretic fx.

Use: angina Px[1], HTN[2] (*for advice on stepped HTN Mx see p. 182*), Raynaud's[3].

CI: cardiogenic shock, clinically significant aortic stenosis, ACS (inc w/in 1 month of MI).

Caution: angina or LVF can worsen (consider stopping drug), ↓BP, DM, BPH, acute porphyria **L/R/H/P/B**.

SE: flushing, headache, ankle oedema, dizziness, ↓BP, palpitations, poly-/nocturia, rash/pruritus, GI upset, weakness, myalgia, arthralgia, gum hyperplasia, rhinitis. Rarely, PU, hepatotoxicity.

Interactions: metab by **P450**. ↑s fx of digoxin, theophylline and tacrolimus. ↓s fx of quinidine. Quinu-/dalfo-pristin, ritonavir and grapefruit juice ↑fx of nifedipine. Rifampicin, phenytoin and carbamazepine ↓fx of nifedipine. Risk of ↓↓BP with α-blockers, β-blockers or Mg^{2+} iv/im.

Dose: 5–20 mg tds po[3]; use long-acting preparations for HTN/angina, as normal-release preparations $\Rightarrow$ erratic BP control and reflex ↑HR, which can worsen IHD (e.g. Adalat LA or Retard and many others with differing fx and doses[SPC/BNF]). NB: ↓dose if severe LF.

NITROFURANTOIN

Antibiotic: only active in urine (no systemic antibacterial fx).

Use: UTIs (but not pyelonephritis).

CI: G6PD deficiency, acute porphyria, **R** (also $\Rightarrow$ ↓activity of drug: it needs to be concentrated in urine), infants <3 yrs old, **P/B**.

Caution: DM, lung disease, ↓Hb, ↓vitamin B, ↓folate, electrolyte imbalance, susceptibility to peripheral neuropathy, **L/E**.

SE: GI upset, pulmonary reactions (inc effusions, fibrosis), peripheral neuropathy, hypersensitivity. Rarely, hepatotoxicity, cholestasis, pancreatitis, arthralgia, alopecia (transient), skin reactions (esp exfoliative dermatitis), blood disorders, BIH.

Dose: 50 mg qds po ($\uparrow$to 100 mg if severe chronic recurrent infection); od nocte if for Px. *Take with food.* Not available iv or im.

NB: can $\Rightarrow$ false-positive urine dipstick for glucose and discolour urine.

NORADRENALINE (= NOREPINEPHRINE)

Vasoconstrictor sympathomimetic: stimulates α-receptors $\Rightarrow$ vasoconstriction.

Use: $\downarrow$BP (unresponsive to other Rx)[1], cardiac arrest[2].

CI: $\uparrow$BP, **P**.

Caution: thrombosis (coronary/mesenteric/peripheral), Prinzmetal's angina, post-MI, $\uparrow T_4$, DM, $\downarrow O_2$, $\uparrow CO_2$, hypovolaemia (uncorrected), **E**.

SE: can $\downarrow$BF to vital organs (esp kidney). Also headache, $\downarrow$HR, arrhythmias, peripheral ischaemia. $\uparrow$BP if over-Rx.

Interactions: 🔔 risk of arrhythmias with halothane and cyclopropane 🔔. Risk of $\uparrow$BP with clonidine, MAOIs and TCAs.

Dose: 80 microgram/ml ivi at 0.16–0.33 ml/min[1] (adjust according to response); 0.5–0.75 ml of 200 microgram/ml solution iv stat[2].

(🔔 NB: *doses given here are for noradrenaline* **acid tartrate**, *not* base 🔔).

NORETHISTERONE

Progestogen (testosterone analogue).

Use: endometriosis[1], dysfunctional uterine bleeding and menorrhagia[2], dysmenorrhoea[3], postponement of menstruation[4].

CI: liver/genital/breast cancers (unless progestogens being used for these conditions), atherosclerosis, undiagnosed vaginal bleeding, acute porphyria, Hx of idiopathic jaundice, severe pruritis, pemphigoid during pregnancy.

Caution: risk of fluid retention, TE disease, DM, depression. **L/H/R**.

SE: $\uparrow$weight, nausea, headache, dizziness, insomnia, drowsiness, breast tenderness, acne, depression, Δ libido, skin reactions, hirsuitism & alopecia.

Dose: 5 mg bd-tds po for ≥4–6 months, commencing on day 5 of cycle (can ↑ to 10 mg bd-tds if spotting occurs, ↓ing when stops)[1]; 5 mg tds po for 10 days for Rx (for Px give 5 mg bd po from day 19–26 of cycle)[2]; 5 mg tds po from day 5–24 for 3–4 cycles[3]; 5 mg tds po starting 3 days prior to expected menstruation onset (bleeding will commence 2–3 days after stopping)[4].

NUROFEN see Ibuprofen; NB: 'over-the-counter' use can ⇒ poor response to HTN and HF Rx.

NYSTATIN

Polyene antifungal.
Use: *Candida* infections: topically for skin/mucous membranes (esp mouth/vagina); po for GI infections (not absorbed).
SE: GI upset (at ↑doses), skin reactions.
Dose: po suspension: 0.5–1 million units qds, usually for 1 wk, for Rx (or 1 million units od for Px) *after food*.

OFLOXACIN 0.3% EYE DROPS/EXOCIN

Topical antibiotic; mostly used for corneal ulcers[1] (only start if corneal Gram stain/cultures taken and specialist not available).
Caution: P/B.
SE: local irritation. Rarely dizziness, headache, numbness, nausea.
Dose: 1 drop 2–4 hourly for 1st 2 days then qds (max 10 days)[1]. See SPC for other uses.

OLANZAPINE/ZYPREXA

'Atypical' antipsychotic: D_1, D_2, D_4 and $5HT_2$ (+ mild muscarinic) antagonist.
Use: schizophrenia[NICE], mania, bipolar Px, acute sedation.
CI: glaucoma (angle closure), **B. If giving im** also acute MI/ACS, ↓↓BP/HR, SSS or recent heart surgery. See also Chlorpromazine.
Caution: drugs that ↑QTc, dementia, cardiovascular disease (esp if Hx of or ↑risk of CVA/TIA), DM*, ↑prostate, Parkinson's, Hx of epilepsy, blood disorders, paralytic ileus. ↑s fx of alcohol, L/R/H/P/E.

SE: sedation, ↑Wt, ankle oedema, Δ LFTs, postural ↓BP (esp initially ∴ titrate up dose slowly). ↑**glucose*** (rarely ☠DM/DKA☠). Also extrapyramidal/anticholinergic fx (see p. 233; often transient) and rarely neuroleptic malignant syndrome and hepatotoxicity.

Monitor: BG* (± HbA$_{1C}$), LFTs, U&Es, FBC, prolactin, Wt, lipids (and CK if neuroleptic malignant syndrome suspected). If giving im closely monitor cardiorespiratory function for ≥4 h post-dose, esp if given other antipsychotic or benzodiazepine.

Interactions: metab by **P450** ∴ many, but most importantly, levels ↓by carbamazepine and smoking. ↑risk of ↓NØ with valproate. Levels may be ↑by ciprofloxacin. ↑risk of CNS toxicity with sibutramine. ↑risk of arrhythmias with drugs that ↑QTc and atomoxetine. ↑risk of ↓BP with general anaesthetics. ↓s fx of anticonvulsants.

Dose: 5–20 mg po daily (preferably nocte to avoid daytime sedation). Available in 'melt' form if ↓compliance/swallowing (as Velotab). Available in quick-acting im form (▼) for acute sedation; give 5–10 mg (2.5–5 mg in elderly) repeating 2 h later if necessary to max total daily dose, inc po doses, of 20 mg (max 3 injections/day for 3 days).

NB: im doses not recommended with im/iv benzodiazepines (↑risk of respiratory depression) which should be given ≥1 h later; if benzodiazepines already given, use with caution and closely monitor cardiorespiratory function.

OLMESARTAN/OLMETEC

Angiotensin II antagonist: see Losartan.

Use: HTN; *for advice on stepped HTN Mx see p. 182*.

CI: biliary obstruction, **P/B**.

Caution/SE/Interactions: see Losartan.

Dose: initially 10 mg od, ↑ing to max 40 mg (20 mg in LF, RF or elderly).

OMEGA-3-ACID ETHYL ESTERS 90/OMACOR

Essential fatty acid combination: 1 g capsule = eicosapentaenoic acid 460 mg and decosahexaenoic acid 380 mg.

Use: Adjunct to diet in type IIb and III ↑TG[1] (with statin) or type IV. Added for 2° prevention w/in 3 months of acute MI[2].

CI: **B**.

Caution: bleeding disorders, anticoagulants, DM **L/P**.

SE: GI; rarer: taste disorder, dry nose, dizziness, hypersensitivity, hepatotoxicity, headache, rash, ↓BP, DM, ↑WBC.

Monitor: LFTs, INR.

Dose: Capsules: 2–4 g od[1]; 1 g od[2]. Take with food.

OMEPRAZOLE/LOSEC

PPI: inhibits H^+/K^+ ATPase of parietal cells ⇒ ↓acid secretion.

Use: PU Rx/Px (esp if on NSAIDs), gastro-oesophageal reflux disease (if symptoms severe or complicated by haemorrhage/ulcers/stricture)[NICE]. Also used for *H. pylori* eradication and ZE syndrome.

Caution: can mask symptoms of gastric Ca, **L/P/B**.

SE: GI upset, headache, dizziness, arthralgia, weakness, skin reactions. Rarely, hepatotoxicity, blood disorders, hypersensitivity.

Interactions: ↓ (and ↑) **P450** ∴ many, most importantly ↑s phenytoin, cilostazol, diazepam, raltegravir and digoxin levels. ↓s fx of ataza-/nelfi-/tipra-navir, mild **W +** .

Dose: 20 mg od po, ↑ing to 40 mg in severe/resistant cases and ↓ing to 10 mg od for maintenance if symptoms stable; 20 mg bd for *H. pylori* eradication regimens (see p. 175). If unable to take po (e.g. perioperatively, ↓GCS, on ITU), give 40 mg iv od either over 5 min or as ivi over 20–30 min. **NB: max dose 20 mg if LF.**

NB: also specialist use iv for acute bleeds. Usually as 8 mg/h ivi for 72 h if endoscopic evidence of PU (prescribed as divided infusions, as drug is unstable). Contact pharmacy ± GI team for advice on indications and exact dosing regimens.

ONDANSETRON

Antiemetic: 5HT$_3$ antagonist: acts on central and GI receptors.

Use: N&V, esp if resistant to other Rx or severe postoperative/chemotherapy-induced.

Caution: GI obstruction (inc subacute), ↑QTc*, **L** (unless mild), **P/B**.

SE: constipation (or diarrhoea), **headache**, sedation, fatigue, dizziness. Rarely seizures, chest pain, ↓BP, Δ LFTs, rash, hypersensitivity.

Interactions: metab by **P450**. Levels ↓by rifampicin, carbamazepine and phenytoin. ↓s fx of tramadol. Avoid with drugs that ↑QTc*.
Dose: 8 mg bd po; 16 mg od pr; 8 mg 2–8-hrly iv/im. Max 24 mg/day usually (8 mg/day if LF). Can also give as ivi at 1 mg/h for max of 24 h. Exact dose and route depends on indication[SPC/BNF].

ORAMORPH Oral morphine solution for severe pain, esp useful for prn or breakthrough pain (see p. 189 for use in palliative care).
Dose: Multiply sc/im morphine dose by 2 to obtain approx equivalent[Oramorph] dose. NB: ↓dose if LF or RF.

Solution mostly commonly used is 10 mg/5 ml, but can be 100 mg/5 ml ∴ *specify strength if prescribing in ml (rather than mg).*

OTOSPORIN Ear drops for otitis externa (esp if bacterial infection suspected): contains antibacterials (neomycin, polymyxin B) and hydrocortisone 1%.
Dose: 3 drops tds/qds.

OXYBUTYNIN

Anticholinergic (selective M_3 antagonist); antispasmodic (↓s bladder muscle contractions).
Use: detrusor instability (also neurogenic bladder instability, nocturnal enuresis).
CI: bladder outflow or GI obstruction, urinary retention, severe UC/ toxic megacolon, glaucoma (narrow angle), MG, **B**.
Caution: ↑prostate, autonomic neuropathy, hiatus hernia (if reflux), ↑T_4, IHD, arrhythmias, porphyria, L/R/H/P/E.
SE: antimuscarinic fx (see p. 233), GI upset, palpitations/↑HR, skin reactions – mostly dose-related and reportedly less severe in MR preparations*.
Dose: initially 5 mg bd/tds po (2.5 mg bd if elderly) ↑ing if required to max of 5 mg qds (bd if elderly). Also available as MR tablet (Lyrinel XL* 5–20 mg od) and transdermal patch (Kentera 36 mg; releases 3.9 mg/day and lasts 3–4 days).

OXYCODONE (HYDROCHLORIDE)/OXYNORM

Opioid for moderate/severe pain (esp in palliative care.)
CI: as fentanyl, plus acute abdomen, delayed gastric emptying, chronic constipation, cor pulmonale, acute porphyria. **L**(if moderate/severe)/**R** (if severe), **P/B**.
Caution: all other conditions where morphine is CI/cautioned.
SE/Interactions: as morphine, but does not interact with baclofen, gabapentin and ritonavir.
Dose: 4–6-hrly po/sc/iv or as sc infusion. NB: 2.5 mg sc/iv = 5 mg po = approx 10 mg morphine po. Available in MR form as OxyContin (12-hrly). Available with naloxone (works locally to ↓GI SEs) as ▼ Targinact (12-hrly). NB: ↓dose if LF, RF or elderly.

OXYTETRACYCLINE

Tetracycline antibiotic: inhibits ribosomal protein synthesis.
Use: acne vulgaris (and rosacea).
CI/Caution/SE/Interactions: as tetracycline, plus caution in porphyria.
Dose: 500 mg bd po (1 h before food or on empty stomach) for ≥16 wks.

PABRINEX

Parenteral (iv or im) vitamins that come as a pair of vials. Vial 1 contains B_1 (thiamine*), B_2 (riboflavin) and B_6 (pyridoxine). Vial 2 contains C (ascorbic acid), nicotinamide and glucose.
Use: Acute vitamin deficiencies (esp thiamine*).
Caution: Rarely ⇒ **anaphylaxis** (esp if given iv too quickly). *Ensure access to resuscitation facilities.*

*See p. 195 for Wernicke's encephalopathy Px/Rx in alcohol withdrawal.

(DISODIUM) PAMIDRONATE

Bisphosphonate: ↓s osteoclastic bone resorption.
Use: ↑Ca^{2+} (esp metastatic: also ↓s pain)[1], Paget's disease[2], myeloma.
CI: **P/B**.

Caution: Hx of thyroid surgery, cardiac disease, **L/R/H**.

SE: 'flu-like symptoms (inc fever, transient pyrexia), **GI upset** (inc haemorrhage), **dizziness/somnolence** (common post-dose*), ↑ (or ↓) BP, seizures, musculoskeletal pain, osteonecrosis of jaw (esp in cancer patients; consider dental examination or preventative Rx – MHRA advice), e'lyte Δs ($\downarrow PO_4$, ↓or $\uparrow K^+$, $\uparrow Na^+$, $\downarrow Mg^{2+}$), RF, blood disorders.

Monitor: e'lytes (inc U&E before each dose), Ca^{2+}, PO_4^-, before starting biphosphonate consider dental check as risk of osteonecrosis of the jaw.

Warn: not to drive/operate machinery immediately after Rx*.

Dose: 15–90 mg ivi according to indication ($\pm Ca^{2+}$ levels[1]). **NB: if RF max rate of ivi 20 mg/h (unless for life-threatening $\uparrow Ca^{2+}$).** *Never given regularly for sustained periods.*

PANTOPRAZOLE

PPI; as omeprazole, but ↓interactions and can ⇒ ↑TGs.

Dose: 20–80 mg mane po (↓ing to 20 mg maintenance if symptoms allow). If unable to take po (e.g. perioperatively, ↓GCS, on ITU), can give 40 mg iv over ≥2 min (or as ivi) od. ↑doses if ZE syndrome[SPC/BNF]. **NB: ↓dose if RF or LF.**

PARACETAMOL

Antipyretic & mild analgesic. Unlike NSAIDs, *has no anti-inflammatory fx.*

Use: mild pain (or moderate/severe in combination with other Rx), pyrexia.

Caution: alcohol dependence, **L** (CI if severe liver disease), **R**.

SE: *all rare:* rash, blood disorders, hepatic (rarely renal) failure – esp if over-Rx/OD (for Mx, see p. 261).

Interactions: may **W** + if prolonged regular use.

Dose: 0.5–1 g po/pr; 1 g (or 15 mg/kg if <50 kg) iv. All doses 4–6 hourly, max 4 g/day. Max 3 g/day iv (▼) in LF, dehydration, chronic alcoholism or chronic malnutrition. Minimum iv dosing interval in RF: 6-hrly. (For children, see Calpol.)

PAROXETINE/SEROXAT

SSRI antidepressant; as fluoxetine, but $\downarrow t_{1/2}$*.

Use: depression[1], other Ψ disorders (social/generalised anxiety disorder[1], PTSD[1], panic disorder[2], OCD[3]).

CI/Caution/SE/Interactions: as fluoxetine, but ↓frequency of agitation/insomnia, although ↑frequency of **antimuscarinic fx** (see p. 233), **extrapyramidal fx** (see p. 236) and **withdrawal fx*** (see p. 235). Avoid if < 18 yrs old as may ↑suicide risk & hostility[SPC]. Also does not ↑carbamazepine levels (but its levels are ↓by carbamazepine) but ↑s galantamine levels. Risk of CNS toxicity if given with tramadol. Avoid if patient enters manic stage. **P**.

Dose: initially 20 mg[1,3] (10 mg[2]) mane, ↑ing if required to max 50 mg[1] or 60 mg[2,3].

NB: ↓dose if RF, LF or elderly.

Stop very slowly as short $t_{1/2}$ ⇒ ↑risk of withdrawal syndrome.

PARVOLEX see Acetylcysteine; antidote for paracetamol poisoning.

PENICILLAMINE

Chelates copper/lead ⇒ ↑elimination (also acts as DMARD): slow onset of action (6–12 wks).

Use: Wilson's disease*, copper/lead poisoning, rarely for rheumatoid arthritis (also autoimmune hepatitis, cystinuria).

CI: SLE, **R** (unless mild when only caution).

Caution: penicillin allergy (can also be penicillamine allergic), taking other nephrotoxic drugs, **P**.

SE: RF (esp immune nephritis ⇒ proteinuria*: stop drug if severe), **blood disorders** (↓Pt, ↓NØ, agranulocytosis, aplastic ↓Hb), **rashes** (inc SJS, pemphigus), **taste Δs**, **GI upset** (esp nausea, but ↓s if taken with food). Can ↑neurological symptoms in Wilson's. Rarely hepatotoxicity, pancreatitis, autoimmune phenomena: poly-/dermato-myositis, Goodpasture's syndrome, lupus-/myasthenia-like syndromes.

Warn: immediately report sore throat, fever, infection, non-specific illness, unexpected bleeding/bruising, purpura, mouth ulcers or rash.

Monitor: FBC, U&Es, urine dipstick ±24-h collection*.

Interactions: ↑risk of agranulocytosis with clozapine. Absorption ↓by antacids and FeSO₄. Can ↓levels of digoxin.
Dose: 125–2000 mg daily^{SPC/BNF} depending on indication. **NB:** consider ↓dose if RF or elderly.

Can ⇒ ↓pyridoxine which often needs supplementing. Consider stopping if fever, lymphadenopathy, ↓Pt/N∅, proteinuria or worsening neuro symptoms. Sensitivity occurs in 10%; can restart with prednisolone – get senior advice.

PENICILLIN G see Benzylpenicillin.

PENICILLIN V see Phenoxymethylpenicillin.

PENTASA see Mesalazine; aminosalicylate for UC, with ↓SEs.

PEPPERMINT OIL

Antispasmodic: direct relaxant of GI smooth muscle.
Use: GI muscle spasm, distension (esp IBS).
SE: perianal irritation, indigestion. Rarely rash or other allergy.
Dose: 1–2 capsules tds, before meals and with water.

PEPTAC Alginate raft-forming oral suspension for acid reflux.
Dose: 10–20 ml after meals and at bedtime (NB: 3 mmol Na⁺/5 ml).

PERINDOPRIL/COVERSYL

ACE-i; see Captopril.
Use: HTN (*for advice on stepped HTN Mx see p. 182*), HF, Px of IHD.
CI/Caution/SE/Monitor/Interactions: as Captopril, plus can ⇒ mood/sleep Δs.
Dose: 2–8 mg od^{SPC/BNF}, starting at 2–4 mg od. NB: consider ↓dose if RF, elderly, taking a diuretic, cardiac decompensation or volume depletion.

PETHIDINE

Opioid; less potent than morphine but quicker action ⇒ ↑euphoria + abuse/dependence potential ∴ not for chronic use e.g. in palliative care.

Use: moderate/severe pain, obstetric and peri-op analgesia.
CI: acute respiratory depression, risk of ileus, ↑ICP/head injury/coma, phaeo.
Caution: any other condition where morphine CI/cautioned.
SE: as morphine, but ↓constipation.
Interactions: as morphine but 🐝 ↑risk of hyperpyrexia/CNS toxicity with **MAOIs** 🐝. Ritonavir ⇒ ↓levels and ↑s toxic metabolites. May ↑serotonergic effects of duloxetine. No known interaction with gabapentin or baclofen.
Dose: 25–100 mg up to 4-hrly im/sc (can give 2-hrly post-op or 1–3-hrly in labour with max 400 mg/24 hrs); 25–50 mg up to 4-hrly slow iv. Rarely used po: 50–150 mg up to 4-hrly. **NB: ↓dose if LF, RF or elderly.**

PHENOBARBITAL (= PHENOBARBITONE)

Barbiturate antiepileptic: potentiates GABA (inhibitory neurotransmitter), antagonises fx of glutamate (excitatory neurotransmitter).
Use: status epilepticus (SEs and interactions limit other uses).
Caution: respiratory depression, acute porphyria, **L/R/P/B/E.**
SE: hepatitis, cholestasis, respiratory depression, sedation, ↓BP, ↓HR, ataxia, skin reactions. Rarely, paradoxical excitement (esp in elderly), blood disorders.
Interactions: ↑**P450** ∴ many, most importantly ↓s levels/fx of aripiprazole, antivirals, carbamazepine, Ca²⁺ antagonists, chloramphenicol, corticosteroids, ciclosporin, eplerenone, mianserin, tacrolimus, telithromycin, posa-/vori-conazole and OCP. Anticonvulsant fx ↓by antipsychotics, TCAs and SSRIs. Avoid with St John's wort. ↑s fx of sodium oxybate. Caution with other sedative drugs (esp benzodiazepines), **W–.**
Dose: total of 10 mg/kg as ivi at 50–100 mg/min (max total 1 g).

PHENOXYMETHYLPENICILLIN (= PENICILLIN V)

As benzylpenicillin (penicillin G) but active orally: used for ENT/skin infections (esp erisipelas), Px of rheumatic fever/*S. pneumoniae* infections (esp post-splenectomy).

Dose: 0.5–1.0 g qds po (take on empty stomach; $\geq$ 1 hr before food or $\geq$ 2 hrs after food).

PHENTOLAMINE

α-Blocker, short-acting.
Use: HTN 2° to phaeo (esp during surgery).
CI: ↓BP, IHD (inc Hx of MI).
Caution: PU/gastritis, asthma, R/P/B/E.
SE: ↓BP, ↑HR, dizziness, weakness, flushing, GI upset, nasal congestion. Rarely, coronary/cerebrovascular occlusion, arrhythmias.
Interactions: see Doxazosin.
Dose: 2–5 mg iv (repeat if necessary).

PHENYLEPHRINE EYE DROPS

Topical sympathomimetic for pupil dilation (commonly used in combination with cyclopentolate or tropicamide).
Caution: cardiovascular disease, ↑HR, ↑T_4, children E.
SE: blurred vision, local irritation, ↑BP, ↑HR, arrhythmias, coronary artery spasm.
Dose: 1 drop. 2.5% drops most common (10% available but ↑risk of ↑BP.

PHENYTOIN

Antiepileptic: blocks Na^+ channels (stabilises neuronal membranes).
Use: all forms of epilepsy[1] (except absence seizures) inc status epilepticus[2].
CI: *if giving iv* (do not apply if po); sinus ↓HR, Stokes–Adams syndrome, SAN block, 2nd-/3rd-degree HB, acute porphyria.
Caution: DM, porphyria ↓BP, L/H/P ($\Rightarrow$ cleft lip/palate, congenital heart disease), B.
SE (acute): *dose-dependent*: **drowsiness** (also confusion/dizziness), **cerebellar fx** (see p. 236), **rash** (common cause of intolerance and rarely $\Rightarrow$ SJS/TEN), N&V, diplopia, dyskinesia (esp orofacial). *If iv, risk of ↓BP, arrhythmias** (esp ↑QTc), **'purple glove syndrome'** (hand damage distal to injection site), CNS/respiratory depression.

SE (chronic): gum hypertrophy, coarse facies, hirsutism, acne, ↓folate (⇒ megaloblastic ↓Hb), Dupuytren's, peripheral neuropathy, rickets, osteomalacia. Rarely, blood disorders, hepatotoxicity, suicidal thoughts/behaviour.

Monitor: FBC**, keep serum levels at 10–20 mg/l (narrow therapeutic index). 💀 If iv, closely monitor BP and ECG* (esp QTc)💀.

Warn: report immediately any rash, mouth ulcers, sore throat, fever, bruising, bleeding.

Interactions: metab by and ↑s **P450** ∴ many; most importantly ↓s fx of OCP, doxycycline, Ca²⁺ antagonists (esp nifedipine), imatinib, lapatinib, ciclosporin, keto-/itra-/posa-conazole, indinavir, quinidine, theophyllines, eplerenone, telithromycin, aripiprazole, mianserin, mirtazapine, paroxetine, TCAs and corticosteroids. Fx ↓by rifampicin, rifabutin, theophyllines, mefloquine, pyrimethamine, sucralfate, antipsychotics, TCAs and St John's wort. Levels ↑by NSAIDs (esp azapropazone), fluoxetine, mi-/flu-/vori-conazole, diltiazem, disulfiram, trimethoprim, cimetidine, esomeprazole, amiodarone, metronidazole, chloramphenicol, clarithromycin, isoniazid, sulphonamides, sulfinpyrazone, topiramate (levels of which are ↓) and ethosuximide. Complex interactions with other antiepileptics^SPC/BNF. **W−** (or rarely **W+**).

Dose: po¹: 150–500 mg/day in 1–2 divided doses^SPC/BNF. iv²: load with 18 mg/kg ivi at max rate of 25–50 mg/min, then maintenance iv doses of approximately 100 mg tds/qds, adjusting to weight, serum levels and clinical response. If available give iv as *fosphenytoin* (NB: doses differ).

NB: ↓dose if LF.

💀 Stop drug if ↓WCC** is severe, worsening or symptomatic 💀.

PHOSPHATE ENEMA

Laxative enemas; ⇒ osmotic H₂O retention ⇒ ↑evacuation.
Use: severe constipation (unresponsive to other Rx).
CI: acute GI disorders.
Caution: if debilitated or neurological disorder, **E**.
SE: local irritation.

Dose: 1 prn.

PHYLLOCONTIN CONTINUS see Aminophylline (MR).
Dose: initially 1 tablet (225 mg) bd po, then ↑ to 2 tablets bd after 1 wk according to serum levels. (Forte tablets of 350 mg used if smoker/other cause of ↓$t_{1/2}$, e.g. interactions with other drugs; see Theophylline.) **NB:** ↓**dose if LF.**

PHYTOMENADIONE

Intravenous vit K_1 for warfarin overdose/poisoning; see p. 211.
Caution: give iv injections slowly. NB: not compative with NaCl **P.**
PICOLAX see Bowel preparations.
Dose: 1 sachet at 8 am and 3 pm the day before GI surgery or Ix.

▼ PIOGLITAZONE/ACTOS

Thiazolidinedione (glitazone) antidiabetic; ↓s peripheral insulin resistance (and, to lesser extent, hepatic gluconeogenesis).
Use: type 2 DM in combination with a sulphonylurea (if metformin not tolerated) *or* metformin (if risk of ↓glucose with sulphonylurea unacceptable) *or* sulphonylurea + metformin (if obese, metabolic syndrome or human insulin unacceptable due to lifestyle/personal issues)[NICE].
CI: ACS (inc Hx of), **H** (inc Hx of), **L/P/B**
Caution: peri-operatively cardiovascular disease. Omit pioglitazone peri-operatively as insulin needed. **R.**
SE: oedema (esp if HTN/CCF), ↓Hb, ↑Wt, GI upset (esp diarrhoea), headache, hypoglycaemia (if also taking sulphonylureas), ↑risk of distal fractures, rarely **hepatotoxicity.**
Monitor: LFTs. ☠*Discontinue if jaundice develops*☠ and for signs of HF.
Interactions: levels ↓by rifampicin and ↑by gemfibrozil.
Dose: initially 15–30 mg od (max 45 mg od)

PIPERACILLIN

Ureidopenicillin: antipseudomonal.
Use: only available with tazobactam* (β-lactamase inhibitor) as Tazocin, reserved for severe infections.

CI/Caution/SE/Interactions: see Benzylpenicillin.
Dose: see Tazocin*.

PIRITON see Chlorphenamine; antihistamine for allergies.

PLAVIX see Clopidogrel; anti-Pt agent for Px of IHD (and CVA).

POTASSIUM TABLETS see Kay-cee-L (syrup 1 mmol/ml),
Sando-K (effervescent 12 mmol/tablet) and Slow-K (MR non-effervescent 8 mmol/tablet, reserved for when syrup/effervescent preparations are inappropriate; avoid if ↓swallow).

PRAMIPEXOLE/MIRAPEXIN
Dopamine agonist (non-ergot derived); use in early Parkinson's ⇒ ↓motor complications (e.g. dyskinesias) but ↓motor performance cf L-dopa.
Use: Parkinson's[1], moderate-severe restless legs syndrome (RLS)[2].
CI: B.
Caution: psychotic disorders, severe cardiovascular disease **R/H/P.**
SE: GI upset, sleepiness (inc sudden onset sleep), ↓BP (inc postural, esp initially), Ψ disorders (esp psychosis and impulse control disorders e.g. gambling and ↑sexuality), amnesia, headache, oedema.
Warn: sleepiness and ↓BP may impair skilled tasks (inc driving). Avoid abrupt withdrawal.
Monitor: ophthalmological testing if visual Δs occur.
Dose: initially 88 microgram tds[1] (or 88 microgram nocte for RLS[2]) ↑ing if tolerated/required to max 1.1 mg tds[1] (or 540 microgram nocte[2]). **NB: doses given for BASE (not SALT) & ↓dose if RF.**

PRAVASTATIN/LIPOSTAT
HMG-CoA reductase inhibitor: 'statin'; ↓s cholesterol/LDL (and TG).
Use/CI/Caution/SE/Monitor: see Simvastatin.
Interactions: ↑risk of myositis (± ↑levels) with ☣ fibrates☠, nicotinic acid, daptomycin, ciclosporin and ery-/clari-thromycin.
Dose: 10–40 mg nocte. **NB: ↓dose if RF** (10 mg if moderate to severe RF).

PREDNISOLONE

Glucocorticoid (and mild mineralocorticoid activity).

Use: anti-inflammatory (e.g. rheumatoid arthritis, IBD, asthma, eczema), immunosuppression (e.g. transplant rejection Px, acute leukaemias), glucocorticoid replacement (e.g. Addison's disease, hypopituitarism).

CI: systemic infections (w/o antibiotic cover).

Caution/SE/Interactions: see p. 225.

Warn: carry steroid card (and avoid close contact with people who have chickenpox/shingles if patient has never had chickenpox).

Dose: usually 2.5–15 mg od po for maintenance. In acute/initial stages, 20–60 mg od often needed (depends on cause and often physician preference), e.g. acute asthma (40 mg od), acute COPD (30 mg od), temporal arteritis (40–60 mg daily). Take with food ($\downarrow Na^+$, $\uparrow K^+$ diet recommended if on long-term Rx). For other causes, consult$^{SPC/BNF}$, pharmacy or local specialist relevant to the disease. Also available as once or twice weekly im injection.

> ☠Warn patient not to stop tablets suddenly (*can* ⇒ *Addisonian crisis*). Requirements may ↑ if intercurrent illness/surgery. Consider Ca/vit D supplements/bisphosphonate to ↓risk of osteoporosis and PPI to ↓risk of GI ulcer☠.

PREGABALIN/LYRICA

Antiepileptic; GABA analogue.

Use: epilepsy (partial seizures w or w/o 2° generalisation), neuropathic pain, generalised anxiety disorder.

CI: B.

Caution: avoid abrupt withdrawal, **H** (if severe) **R/P/E**.

SE: neuro-Ψ disturbance; esp **somnolence/dizziness** (⇒ falls in elderly), confusion, visual Δ (esp blurred vision), mood ↑ or ↓ (and *possibly* suicidal ideation/behaviour[†]), ↓libido, sexual dysfunction and vertigo. Also GI upset, ↑appetite/Wt, oedema and dry mouth. Rarely HF (esp if elderly and/or CVS disease).

Warn: seek medical advice if ↑suicidality or mood ↓s[†]. Don't stop abruptly as can ⇒ withdrawal fx* (insomnia, headache, N&D, 'flu-like symptoms, pain, sweating, dizziness, pain).
Dose: 50–600 mg/day po in 2–3 divided doses[SPC/BNF]. **NB: stop over ≥1wk* and ↓dose if RF.**

PROCHLORPERAZINE/STEMETIL

Antiemetic: DA antagonist (phenothiazine ∴ also antipsychotic, but now rarely used for this).
Use: N&V (inc labyrinthine disorders).
CI/Caution/SE/Monitor/Warn/Interactions: as chlorpromazine, but CI are relative and ⇒ ↓sedation. NB: can ⇒ **extrapyramidal fx** (esp if elderly/debilitated); see p. 236.
Dose: *po:* acutely 20 mg, then 10 mg 2 h later (5–10 mg bd/tds for Px and labyrinthine disorders); **im:** 12.5 mg, then po doses 6 h later; *pr:* 25 mg then po doses 6 h later (5 mg tds pr for migraine). Available as quick-dissolving 3-mg tablets to be placed under lip (Buccastem); give 1–2 bd. **NB: ↓dose if RF.**

PROCYCLIDINE

Antimuscarinic: ↓s cholinergic to dopaminergic ratio in extrapyramidal syndromes ⇒ ↓tremor/rigidity. No fx on bradykinesia (or tardive dyskinesia; may even worsen).
Use: extrapyramidal symptoms (e.g. Parkinsonism), esp if drug-induced[1] (e.g. antipsychotics; see p. 236).
CI: urinary retention (if untreated), glaucoma* (angle-closure), GI obstruction, MG.
Caution: cardiovascular disease, ↑prostate, tardive dyskinesia, **L/R/H/P/B/E.**
SE: antimuscarinic fx (see p. 233), Ψ disturbances, euphoria (can be drug of abuse), glaucoma*.
Warn: can ↓ability at driving/skilled tasks.
Dose: 2.5 mg tds po prn[1] (↑if necessary to max of 10 mg tds); 5–10 mg im/iv if acute dystonia or oculogyric crisis.

NB: do not stop suddenly: can ⇒ rebound muscarinic fx.

PROMETHAZINE

Sedating antihistamine.

Use: insomnia[1] (see p. 230). Also used iv/im for anaphylaxis and po for symptom relief in chronic allergies.

CI: CNS depression/coma, MAOI w/in 14 days.

Caution: urinary retention, ↑prostate, glaucoma, epilepsy, IHD, asthma, porphyria, pyloroduodenal obstruction, **R** (↓dose), **L** (avoid if severe)/**P/B/E**.

SE: antimuscarinic fx (see p. 233), **hangover sedation**, headache.

Warn: can ↓ability at driving/skilled tasks.

Interactions: ↑s fx of anticholinergics, TCAs and sedatives/hypnotics.

Dose: 25 mg nocte[1] (can ↑dose to 50 mg).

PROPRANOLOL

β-Blocker (non-selective): $β_1$ ⇒ ↓HR and ↓contractility, $β_2$ ⇒ vasodilation (and bronchoconstriction and glucose release from liver). Also blocks fx of catecholamines, ↓s renin production, slows SAN/AVN conduction.

Use: HTN[1] (*for advice on stepped HTN Mx see p. 182*), IHD (angina Rx[2], MI Px[3]), portal HTN[4] (Px of variceal bleed; NB: *may worsen liver function*), essential tremor[5], Px of migraine[6], anxiety[7], ↑T (symptom relief[8], thyroid storm[9]), arrhythmias[8] (inc severe[9]).

CI: **asthma/Hx of bronchospasm, peripheral arterial disease** (if severe), Prinzmetal's angina, severe ↓HR or ↓BP, SSS, 2nd-/3rd-degree HB, cardiogenic shock, metabolic acidosis, phaeo (unless used specifically with α-blockers), **H** (if uncontrolled).

Caution: COPD, 1st-degree HB, DM*, MG, Hx of hypersensitivity (may ↑ to *all* allergens), **L/R/P/B**.

SE: ↓HR, ↓BP, HF, **peripheral vasoconstriction** (⇒ cold extremities, worsening of claudication/Raynaud's), **fatigue, depression, sleep disturbance** (inc nightmares), hyperglycaemia (and **↓sympathetic response to hypoglycaemia***), GI upset. Rarely, conduction/blood disorders.

Interactions: ☠ verapamil and diltiazem ⇒ risk of HB and ↓HR ☠. Risk of ↓BP and HF with nifedipine. Risk of ↓BP with α-blockers. ↑s risk of bupiva-/lido-caine toxicity. ↑s risk of AV block, myocardial depression and ↓HR with amiodarone, flecainide. Levels of both drugs can ↑with chlorpromazine. Risk of ↑BP with moxisylyte. Risk of ↑BP (and ↓HR) with dobutamine, adrenaline and noradrenaline. Risk of withdrawal ↑BP with clonidine (stop β-blocker before slowly ↓ing clonidine). ↑level of both chlorpromazine and propranolol if given together.

Dose: 80–160 mg bd po[1]; 40–120 mg bd po[2]; 40 mg qds for 2–3 days, then 80 mg bd po[3] (start 5–21 days post-MI); 40 mg bd po[4] (↑dose if necessary); 40 mg bd/tds po[5,6]; 40 mg od po[7] (↑dose to tds if necessary); 10–40 mg tds/qds[8]; 1 mg iv over 1 min[9] repeating every 2 min if required, to max total 10 mg (or 5 mg in anaesthesia).

NB: ↓po dose in LF and ↓initial dose in RF. Withdraw slowly (esp in angina); if not can ⇒ rebound ↑of symptoms.

PROPYLTHIOURACIL

Thionamide antithyroid (peroxidase inhibitor): ↓s I⁻ ⇒ I₂ ↓s and ∴ ↓T₃/₄ production, as carbimazole does, but also ↓s peripheral T₄ to T₃ conversion. Possible immunosuppressant fx.

Use: ↑T₄ (2nd-line in the UK; if carbimazole not tolerated).

Caution: L/R, P/B (can cause fetal/neonatal goitre/ ↓T₄ ∴ use min dose and monitor neonatal development closely; 'block-and-replace' regimen ∴ not suitable as high doses used for this).

SE: blood disorders (esp ☠ agranulocytosis ☠ stop drug if occurs), skin reactions (esp urticaria, rarely cutaneous vasculitis/lupus), fever. Rarely hepatotoxicity, nephritis.

Warn: patient to report symptoms of infection (esp sore throat) or of liver disease (e.g. anorexia, N&V, jaundice, pruritis), & signs of LF (explain symptoms).

Monitor: FBC, LFTs, clotting.

Dose: 200–400 mg po in divided doses until euthyroid, then ↓ to maintenance dose of 50–150 mg od. NB: ↓dose if LF or RF.

PROSCAR see Finasteride; antiandrogen for BPH (and baldness).

PROTAMINE (SULPHATE)

Protein (basic) that binds heparin (acidic).

Use: reversal of heparin (or LMWH) following over-Rx/OD or after temporary anticoagulation for extracorporeal circuits (e.g. cardio-pulmonary bypass, haemodialysis).

Caution: ↑risk of hypersensitivity reaction if: (1) vasectomy, (2) infertile man, (3) allergy to fish.

SE: ↓BP, ↓HR, N&V, flushing, dyspnoea. Rarely pulmonary oedema, hypertension, **hypersensitivity reactions**.

Dose: 1 mg per 80–100 units of heparin to be reversed (max 50 mg) iv/ivi at rate ≤ 5 mg/min; exact regimen depends on whether reversing heparin or LMWH and whether given iv or sc^BNF/SPC. NB: $t_{1/2}$ of iv heparin is short; ↓doses of protamine if giving to reverse iv heparin >15 min after last dose – see SPC.

> Max total dose 50 mg: ☠ *high doses can* ⇒ *anticoagulant fx!* ☠

PROXYMETHACAINE

Topical anaesthetic (lasts 20 min).

Use: eye examination (if painful eye or checking IOP).

SE: corneal epithelial shedding.

Dose: 1 drop prn (not for prolonged treatment).

PROZAC see Fluoxetine; SSRI antidepressant.

PULMICORT see Budesonide; inh steroid for asthma. 50, 100, 200 or 400 microgram/puff. ▼ Aerosol (not other preparations).

PYRAZINAMIDE

Antibiotic: 'cidal' only against intracellular and dividing mycobacteria (e.g. TB). Good CSF penetration*.

Use: TB Rx (for initial phase, see p. 175), TB meningitis*.

CI: acute porphyria, **L** (if severe, otherwise caution).

Caution: DM, gout (avoid in acute attacks), **P**.

SE: hepatotoxicity**, ↑urate, GI upset (inc N&V), dysuria, interstitial nephritis, **arthr-/my-algia**, sideroblastic ↓Hb, ↓Pt, rash (and photosensitivity).

Monitor: LFTs**.

Warn: patients and carers to stop drug and seek urgent medical attention if signs of LF (explain symptoms).

Dose: up to 2 g daily usually given as part of combination product (500 mg tablets of just pyrazinamide available, but unlicensed)–exact dose varies according to Wt and whether Rx is 'supervised' or not[SPC/BNF].

PYRIDOSTIGMINE

Anticholinesterase: inhibits cholinesterase at neuromuscular junction ⇒ ↑ACh ⇒ ↑neuromuscular transmission.

Use: myasthenia gravis.

CI: GI/urinary obstruction.

Caution: asthma, recent MI, ↓HR/BP, arrhythmias, vagotonia, ↑T, PU, epilepsy, Parkinsonism, R/P/B/E.

SE: cholinergic fx (see p. 233) – esp if xs Rx/OD, where ↓BP, bronchoconstriction and (confusingly) weakness can also occur (= cholinergic crisis*); ↑secretions (sweat/saliva/tears) and miosis are good clues** of xs ACh.

Interactions: fx ↓d by **aminoglycosides** (e.g. gentamicin), **poly-mixins**, clindamycin, lithium, quinidine, chloroquine, propranolol and procainamide. ↑s fx of suxamethonium.

Dose: 30–120 mg po up to qds (can ↑to max total 1.2 g/24 h; if possible give <450 mg/24 h to avoid receptor downregulation).

NB: ↓dose if RF.

> ↑ing weakness can be due to *cholinergic crisis** as well as MG exacerbation; if unsure which is responsible**, get senior help (esp if ↓respiratory function) before giving Rx, as the wrong choice can be fatal!

QUETIAPINE/SEROQUEL

Atypical (2nd generation) antipsychotic.

Use: schizophrenia[1], mania[2], depression in bipolar disorder[3].
Off-licence use for psychosis/behavioural disorders (esp in dementias, but use of antipsychotics in dementia generally not recommended).

CI: B.

Caution: cardiovascular disease, Hx of epilepsy, drugs that ↑QTc, **L/R/E/P**.

SE/Interactions/Warn/Monitor: as olanzapine but therapeutic doses are initially sedating and ↓BP requiring ∴ start with ↓dose*. Also levels ↑by ery-/clari-thromycin.

Dose: *Needs titration* (*see SPC/BNF*): initially 25 mg bd ↑ing daily to max 750 mg/day[1]; initially 50 mg bd ↑ing daily to max 800 mg/day[2]; initially 50 mg od ↑ing daily to max 600 mg/day[3]. If RF, LF or elderly start at 25 mg od ↑ing less frequently. Available in MR form (▼ Seroquel XL); initially 300 mg od then 600 mg od the next day[2], then adjust to response (if giving for depression[3] or if RF, LF or elderly start at 50 mg od then ↑cautiously[SPC/BNF]).

QUININE

Antimalarial: kills bloodborne schizonts.
Use: malaria Rx[1] (esp falciparum), nocturnal leg cramps[2].
CI: optic neuritis, tinnitus, haemoglobinuria, MG.
Caution: cardiac disease (inc conduction dfx, AF, HB), G6PD deficiency, **H/P/E**.
SE: visual Δs (inc temporary blindness, esp in OD), tinnitus (and vertigo/deafness), GI upset, headache, rash/flushing, hypersensitivity, confusion, hypoglycaemia*. Rarely blood disorders, AKI, cardiovascular fx (can ⇒ severe ↓BP in OD).
Monitor: blood glucose*, ECG (if elderly) and e'lytes (if given iv).
Interactions: ↑s levels of flecainide and digoxin. ↑s risk of arrhythmias with pimozide, moxifloxacin and amiodarone. ↑risk of seizures with mefloquine. Avoid artemether/lumefantrine.
Dose: 200–300 mg nocte po as quinine *sulphate*[2]. For malaria Rx, see p. 178 (NB: ↓iv maintenance dose if RF).

RABEPRAZOLE/PARIET

PPI; as omeprazole, but ↓interactions[BNF/SPC].
Dose: 20 mg od (↓to 10 mg od for maintenance). Max 120 mg/day (depending on indication).

RAMIPRIL/TRITACE

ACE-i; see Captopril.

Use: HTN[1] (*for advice on stepped HTN Mx see p. 182*), HF[2], Px post-MI[3]. Also Px of cardiovascular disease (if age > 55 years and at risk)[4].

CI/Caution/SE/Monitor/Interactions: as captopril.

Dose: initially 1.25 mg od (↑ing slowly to max of 10 mg daily)[1,2]; initially 2.5 mg bd then ↑to 5.0 mg bd after 2 days[3] (start 3–10 days post-MI) then maintenance 2.5–5 mg bd; initially 2.5 mg od (↑ing to 10 mg)[4].

NB: ↓dose if RF.

RANITIDINE/ZANTAC

H_2 antagonist ⇒ ↓parietal cell H^+ secretion.

Use: PU (Px if on long-term high dose NSAIDs[1], chronic Rx[2], a cute Rx[3]), reflux oesophagitis.

Caution: acute porphyria, **L/R/P/B**. ☠ *May mask symptoms of gastric cancer* ☠.

SE: *all rare*: GI upset (esp diarrhoea), dizziness, confusion, fatigue, blurred vision, headache, Δ LFTs (rarely hepatitis), rash. Very rarely arrhythmias (esp if given iv), hypersensitivity, blood disorders.

Dose: initially 150 mg bd po (or 300 mg nocte)[1,2], ↑ing to 600 mg/day if necessary but try to ↓ to 150 mg nocte for maintenance; 50 mg tds/qds iv[3] (or im/ivi[SPC/BNF]).

NB: ↓dose if RF.

REOPRO see Abciximab; antiplatelet agent for MI/ACS.

RETEPLASE (= r-PA).

Recombinant plasminogen activator: thrombolytic.

Use/CI/Caution/SE: see Alteplase and p. 215 but only for Rx of AMI (i.e. not for CVA/other use).

Dose: 10 units as slow iv injection over ≤2 min, repeating after 30 min.

Concurrent unfractionated iv heparin needed for 48 h; see p. 215.

RIFABUTIN

Rifamycin antibiotic; see Rifampicin.

Use: TB: Rx of pulmonary TB[1] and non-tuberculous mycobacterial disease[2]. Also Px of *Mycobacterium avium* [3] (if HIV with ↓CD4).

CI/Caution/SE/Warn/Monitor/Interactions: as rifampicin, plus levels ↑ by macrolides, triazoles, imidazoles and antivirals (⇒ ↑risk of uveitis; ↓rifabutin dose) and ↓s carbamazepine levels.

Dose: 150–450 mg od[1]; 450–600 mg od[2]; 300 mg od[3]. **NB:** ↓dose if LF or RF.

RIFAMPICIN

Rifamycin antibiotic: 'cidal' ⇒ ↓RNA synthesis.

Use: TB Rx, *N. meningitides* (meningococcal)/*H. influenzae* (type b) meningitis Px. Rarely for *Legionella/Brucella/Staphylococcus* infections.

CI: jaundice, are concurrently receiving saquinavir/ritonavir therapy, hypersensitivity to rifamycins or excipients.

Caution: acute porphyria, **L/R/P/B**.

SE: **hepatotoxicity**, GI upset (inc AAC), headache, fever, 'flu-like symptoms (esp if intermittent use), orange/red body secretions*, SOB, blood disorders, skin reactions, shock, AKI.

Warn: of symptoms/signs of liver disease; report jaundice/persistent N&V/malaise immediately. Warn about secretions.*

Monitor: LFTs, FBC (and U&Es if dose >600 mg/day).

Interactions: ↑**P450** ∴ many; most importantly ↓s fx of OCP**, lamotrigine, phenytoin, sulphonylureas, rosiglitazone, tolbutamide, chlorpropamide, atovaquone, keto-/flu-itra-/.posa-/vori-conazole, antivirals, telithromycin, nevirapine, ciclosporin, siro-/tacro-limus, imatinib, corticosteroids, haloperidol, aripiprazole, disopyramide, quinidine, mefloquine, bosentan, propafenone, eplerenone and Ca^{2+} antagonists. **W−**.

Dose: for TB Rx, see p. 175; for other indications see SPC/BNF. (NB: well absorbed po; give iv *only* if ↓swallow.) **NB:** ↓dose if LF or RF.

Other contraception** needed during Rx.

RIFATER Combination preparation of rifampicin, isoniazid and pyrazinamide for 1st 2 months of TB Rx ($\Rightarrow$ $\downarrow$bacterial load/infectiousness until sensitivities known); see p. 175.

RISEDRONATE

Bisphosphonate: $\downarrow$s osteoclastic bone resorption.

Use: osteoporosis (Px[1]/Rx[2], esp if postmenopausal or steroid - induced), Paget's disease[3].

CI: $\downarrow$Ca^{2+}, **R** (if eGFR <30 ml/min), **P/B.**

Caution: delayed GI transit/emptying (esp oesophageal abnormal- ities). Correct Ca^{2+} and other bone/mineral metabolism Δ (e.g. vit D and PTH function) before Rx, dental procedures in patients at risk of osteonecrosis of the jaw (e.g. chemotherapy).

SE: GI upset, bone/joint/muscle pain, headache, rash, HTN. Rarely chest pain, oedema, $\downarrow$Wt, apnoea, bronchitis, sinusitis, glossitis, nocturia, infections (esp UTIs), amblyopia, iritis, dry eyes/ corneal lesions, tinnitus and oesophageal stricture/inflammation/ ulcer*, osteonecrosis of the jaw.

Warn: of symptoms of oesophageal irritation and if develop to stop tablets/seek medical attention. Must swallow tablets whole with full glass of water on an empty stomach $\geq$30 min before, and stay upright until, breakfast*.

Interactions: Ca^{2+}-containing products (inc milk) and antacids ($\Rightarrow$ $\downarrow$absorption) $\therefore$ separate doses as much as possible from risedronate. Also avoid iron and mineral suplements.

Dose: 5 mg od[1,2] (or 1 × 35-mg tablet/week as Actonel Once a Week[2]); 30 mg daily for 2 months[3].

▼ RISPERIDONE/RISPERDAL

'Atypical' antipsychotic: similar to olanzapine ($\Rightarrow$ $\downarrow$extrapyramidal fx cf 'typical' antipsychotics, esp tardivedyskinesia).

Use: psychosis/schizophrenia (acute and chronic)[NICE], mania & short term Rx (<6 wks) of persistent aggression unresponsive to non-pharmacological Rx in Alzheimer's.

CI: phenylketonuria (only if Quicklet form used), **B**.
Caution/SE: similar to olanzapine but ⇒↓sedation, ↑hypotension
(esp initially: ↑dose slowly* and consider retitrating if many doses
missed), ↓hyperglycaemia and slightly ↑extrapyramidal fx.
Interactions: levels may be ↓by carbamazepine and ↑by ritonavir,
fluoxetine and paroxetine. ↑risk of CNS toxicity with sibutramine.
↑mortality rate in elderly if taking furosemide. ↑risk of arrhythmias
with drugs that↑QTc and atomoxetine. ↑risk of ↓BP with general-
anaesthetics. ↓s fx of anticonvulsants.
Dose: initially 2 mg od titrating up if necessary, generally to 4–6 mg od
(if elderly initially 0.5 mg bd titrating up if required to max 2 mg bd po).
Also available as liquid or quick dissolving 1, 2, 3, or 4 mg tablets
('Quicklets') and as long-acting im 2-wkly injections ('Consta' ▼) for
↑compliance.
NB: ↓dose if LF or RF.

RITUXIMAB/MABTHERA

Monoclonal Ab against B lymphocytes (CD20 +).
Use: Various B cell non-Hodgkin's lymphoma[1] (many indications for
Diffuse Large B cell Lymphoma and Follicular Lymphoma[NICE]), RA[2]
(in combination with methotrexate, in severe active cases with
inadequate response to DMARDs, inc ≥1 TNF-α inhibitor[NICE]), SLE,
vasculitis, CLL[NICE].
CI: active severe infections, hypersensivity to active substances or
excipients, **B**.
Caution: IHD, if already on othercardiotoxic/cytotoxic drugs, with
active or chronic infections (e.g. hepatitis B), **H** (avoid if severe and
giving for RA)/**P**.
SE: ☠infusion hypersensitivity/cytokine release syndrome* (mainly
during 1st infusion: fever, chills, arrhythmias, ARDS and allergic
reactions)☠, tumour lysis syndrome, pancytopenia, ↓BP, ↑risk of P
ML,↑infections.
Warn: withhold antihypertensive drugs 12 h prior to ivi. Remember
to give patient alert card.
Monitor: BP, neurological function (P ML), FBC.

Dose: seek expert advice and product literature for dose/rate[1], 1 g ivi initially and repeat once after 2 wks[2(see SPC/BNF)].

☠ Only give if full resuscitation facilities available. Interrupt ivi for severe reactions* and institute supportive care measures.

RIVASTIGMINE/EXELON

Acetylcholinesterase inhibitor that acts centrally (crosses BBB): replenishes ACh, which is ↓d in certain dementias.
Use: Alzheimer's disease[NICE] & Parkinson's disease dementia.
CI: L (if severe, otherwise caution), **B**.
Caution: conduction defects (esp SSS), PU susceptibility, Hx of COPD/asthma/seizures, bladder outflow obstruction, **R/P**.
SE: cholinergic fx (see p. 233), **GI upset** (esp nausea initially), **headache**, **dizziness**, behavioural/Ψreactions. Rarely GI haemorrhage, ↓HR, AV block, angina, seizures, rash.
Monitor: weight
Dose: 1.5 mg bd po initially (↑ing slowly to 3–6 mg bd: specialist review needed for clinical response and tolerance). Available as daily sc patch releasing 4.6 mg or 9.5 mg/24 h. Continue only if MMSE remains 10–20[NICE].

NB: If > several days doses missed retitration of dose required.

RIZATRIPTAN/MAXALT

$5HT_{1B/1D}$ agonist for acute migraine.
Use/CI/Caution/SE/Interactions: see Sumatriptan.
Dose: 10 mg po (can repeat after ≥ 2 h if responded then recurs). Max 20 mg/24 h. **NB:** give 5 mg doses if RF or LF (and avoid if either severe).

ROPINIROLE/REQUIP[1] or ADARTREL[2]

Dopamine agonist (non-ergot derived); use in early Parkinson's ⇒ ↓motor complications (e.g. dyskinesias) but ↓motor performance cf L-dopa. Also adjunctive use in Parkinson's with motor fluctuations.
Use: Parkinson's[1], moderate-severe restless legs syndrome (RLS)[2].

CI: P/B.

Caution: major psychotic disorders, severe cardiovascular disease **L/R**.

SE: GI upset, sleepiness (inc sudden onset sleep), ↓BP (inc postural, esp initially), Ψ disorders (esp psychosis and impulse control disorders, e.g. gambling and ↑sexuality), confusion, leg oedema, paradoxical worsening of restless legs syndrome symptoms or early morning rebound (may need to withdraw or reduce dose).

Warn: sleepiness and ↓BP may impair skilled tasks (inc driving). Avoid abrupt withdrawal.

Dose: initially 250 microgram tds[1] (or 250 microgram nocte for RLS[2]) ↑ing if tolerated/required to max 8 mg tds[1] (or 4 mg nocte for RLS[2]). Available in MR preparation (Requip XL) 2–24 mg od[1].

ROSUVASTATIN/CRESTOR

HMG-Co A reductase inhibitor; 'statin' to ↓cholesterol (and TG).

Use/CI/Caution/SE: as simvastatin, but safe in porphyria, can ⇒ proteinuria (and rarely haematuria) and avoid if severe RF.

Interactions: ↑risk of myositis with 💀 **fibrates** and ciclosporin 💀, daptomycin, protease inhibitors and nicotinic acid. Levels ↓ by antacids. Mild **W +**.

Dose: initially 5–10 mg od. If necessary ↑ to 20 mg after ≥4 wks (if not of Asian origin or risk factors for myopathy/rhabdomyolysis, can ↑ to 40 mg after further 4 wks). **NB:** ↓dose if RF, Asian origin or other ↑risk factor for myopathy.

(r)tPA (Recombinant) tissue-type plasminogen activator; see Alteplase.

SALBUTAMOL

β2 Agonist, short-acting: dilates bronchial smooth muscle (and endometrium). Also inhibits mast-cell mediator release.

Use: chronic[1] and acute[2] asthma. Rarely ↑K^+ (give nebs prn), premature labour (iv).

Caution: cardiovascular disease (esp arrhythmias*, susceptibility
to ↑QTc, HTN), DM (can ⇒ DKA, esp if iv ∴ monitor GBGs),
↑T₄, **P/B**.
SE: *neurological*: fine tremor, headache, nervousness, behavioural/sleep
Δs (esp in children); *CVS*: ↑HR, palpitations/arrhythmias (esp if iv),
↑QTc*; *other*: ↓K⁺, muscle cramps. Rarely hypersensitivity, **para-
doxical bronchospasm**. Prolonged Rx ⇒ small↑risk of glaucoma.
Monitor: K⁺ and glucose (esp if ↑ or iv doses).
Interactions: iv salbutamol ⇒ ↑risk of↓↓BP with methyldopa.
Dose: 100–200 microgram (aerosol) or 200–400 microgram (powder)
inh prn up to qds¹; 2.5–5 mg qds 4-hrlyneb². If life - threatening
(see p. 247), can ↑nebs up to every15 min or give as ivi (initially
5 microgram/min, then up to 20 microgram/min according to response).

SALMETEROL/SEREVENT

Bronchodilator: long-acting β₂ agonist(LABA).
Use: 1st choice add-on for asthma Rx (on top of short-acting β₂
agonist and in hsteroids; see BTS guidelines, p. 186). *Not for acute Rx!*
Caution/SE/Monitor: as salbutamol.
Dose: 50–100 microgram bd inh.

SALOFALK see Mesalazine; 'new' aminosalicylate for UC (↓SEs).

SANDOCAL Calcium supplement; available in'400' (400 mg calcium
= 10 mmol Ca²⁺) or '1000' (1 g calcium = 25 mmol Ca²⁺)
effervescent tablets.

SANDO-K
Effervescentoral KCl (12 mmol K⁺/tablet).
Use: ↓K⁺.
CI: K⁺ > 5.0 mmol/l, **R** (if severe, otherwise caution).
Caution: GI ulcer/stricture, hiatus hernia, taking other drugs that ↑K⁺.
SE: N&V, GI ulceration.
Dose: according to serum K⁺: start with 2–4 tablets/day if diet
normal. Take with food. **NB:** ↓**dose in RF/elderly** (↑ if
established ↓K⁺).

SENNA/SENOKOT

Stimulant laxative; takes 8–12 h to work.
Use: constipation.
CI: GI obstruction.
Caution: P (try bulk forming or osmotic laxative 1st).
SE: GI cramps. If chronic use atonic non-functioning colon, $\downarrow K^+$.
Dose: 2 tablets nocte (can $\uparrow$ to 4 tablets nocte). Available as syrup.

SEPTRIN see Co-trimoxazole (sulfamethoxazole + trimethoprim).

SERC see Betahistine; histamine analogue for vestibular disorders.

SERETIDE Combination asthma or COPD inhaler with
possible synergistic action: long-acting β_2 agonist (LABA) salmeterol
50 microgram (Accuhaler) or 25 microgram (Evohaler) + fluticasone
(steroid) in varying quantities (50, 100, 125, 250 or 500 microgram/
puff). Note different devices have different licensed indications.

SEROXAT see Paroxetine; SSRI antidepressant.

SERTRALINE/LUSTRAL

SSRI antidepressant; also increases dopamine levels; see Fluoxetine.
Use: depression (also PTSD in women, OCD, social anxiety disorder
& panic disorder). Relatively good safety record in pregnancy and
breast-feeding.
CI/Caution/SE/Warn/Interactions: as fluoxetine, but $\downarrow$incidence of
agitation/insomnia, doesn't$\uparrow$carbamazepine/phenytoin levels, but does
$\uparrow$pimozide levels.
Dose: initially 50 mg od, $\uparrow$ing in 50 mg increments over several weeks to max
daily dose 200 mg (if > 100 mg/day, must be divided into at least 2 doses).
NB: $\downarrow$**dose if LF.**

SEVELAMER/RENAGEL

PO_4^- binding agent; contains no Al/Ca^{2+} $\therefore$ no risk of$\uparrow$ing Al/Ca^{2+}
(which can occur with other drugs, esp if on dialysis). Also $\downarrow$s
cholesterol.

Use: ↑PO_4 (if on dialysis).

CI: GI obstruction.

Caution: GI disorders, **P/B**.

SE: GI upset, ↓ (or ↑) BP, headache.

Interactions: can ↓ plasma levels of ciprofloxacin and immuno-suppressants used in renal transplant patients.

Dose: initially 800–1600 mg tds po, then adjust to response[SPC/BNF].

SEVREDOL Morphine (sulphate) tablets (10, 20 or 50 mg).

Dose: see Oramorph.

SILDENAFIL/VIAGRA or REVATIO (▼)

Phosphodiesterase type-5 inhibitor: ↑s local fx of NO (⇒ ↑smooth-muscle relaxation ∴ ↑blood flow into corpus cavernosum).

Use: erectile dysfunction[1], pulmonary artery hypertension[2] (and digital ulceration under specialist supervision).

CI: recent CVA/MI/ACS, ↓BP (systolic <90 mmHg), hereditary degenerative retinal disorders, Hx of non-arteritic anterior ischaemic optic neuropathy and conditions where vasodilation/sexual activity inadvisable. **L/H** (if either severe).

Caution: cardiovascular disease, LV outflow obstruction, bleeding disorders (inc active PU), anatomical deformation of penis, predis-position to prolonged erection (e.g. multiple myeloma/leukaemias/sickle cell disease), **R/P/B**.

SE: headache, flushing, GI upset, dizziness, visual disturbances, nasal congestion, hypersensitivity reactions. Rarely, serious cardiovascular events, priapism and painful red eyes.

Interactions: ☠Nitrates (e.g.GTN/ISMN/ISDN) and nicorandil can ↓↓BP ∴ never give together☠. Antivirals (esp rito-/ataza-/indi-navir) ↑its levels. ↑s hypotensive fx of α-blockers; avoid concomitant use. Levels ↑by keto-/itra-conazole

Dose: initially 50 mg approx 1 h before sexual activity[1], adjusting to response (1 dose per 24 h, max 100 mg per dose); 20 mg tds[2]. **NB:** ↓dose if RF or LF.

SIMVASTATIN/ZOCOR

HMG-CoA reductase inhibitor ('statin'): ⇒ ↓cholesterol(↓s synthesis), ↓LDL (↑s uptake), mildly ↓s TG.

Use: ↑cholesterol, Px of atherosclerotic disease: IHD (inc 1° prevention), CVA, PVD.

CI: acute porphyria, **L** (inc active liver disease or ΔLFTs), **P** (contraception required during, and for 1 month after, Rx), **B**.

Caution: ↓T$_4$, alcohol abuse, Hx of liver disease, **R** (if severe).

SE: hepatitis and **myositis*** (both rare but important), headache, GI upset, rash. Rarely pancreatitis, hypersensitivity.

Monitor: LFTs (and CK if symptoms develop*).

Interactions: ↑risk of myositis (± ↑levels) with ☠ **fibrates**☠, clari-/ery-/teli-thromycin, itra-/keto-/mi-/posa-conazole, ciclosporin, **protease inhibitors**, nicotinic acid, fusidic acid, colchicine, danazol, amiodarone, verapamil, diltiazem and grapefruit juice. Mild **W** + .

Dose: 10–80 mg nocte (usually start at 10–20 mg$^{SPC/BNF}$) ↑ing at intervals ≥ 4 wks. ↓max dose if significant drug interactions$^{SPC/BNF}$. **NB:** ↓dose if RF or other ↑risk factor for myositis*.

> ☠ Myositis* can rarely ⇒**rhabdomyolysis**; ↑risk if ↓T$_4$, RF or taking drugs that ↑levels/risk of myositis (see above)☠.

SINEMET see Co-careldopa; L-dopa for Parkinson's.

SLOW-K

Slow-release (non-effervescent) oral KCl (8 mmolK$^+$/tablet).

Use: ↓K$^+$ where liquid/effervescent tablets inappropriate.

CI/Caution/SE: as Sando-K, plus caution if ↓swallow.

Dose: according to serum K$^+$: average 3–6 tablets/day. **NB:** ↓dose if RF (and caution if taking other drugs that ↑K$^+$).

SODIUM BICARBONATE iv

Alkalinising agent.

Use: TCA overdose with ECG Δs; cardiac arrest* (only if due to ↑K$^+$ or TCAs), rarely for severe metabolic acidosis due to xs bicarbonate loss.

SE: paradoxical intracellular acidosis, negative inotrope, ↓s O$_2$ delivery (O$_2$ saturation curve shift), ↓K$^+$, ↑Na$^+$, ↑serum osmolality.

Dose: iv: available in 1.26%, 4.2% and 8.4% solutions; in cardiac arrest* give 50 mmol (50 ml of 8.4% solution) repeating if necessary. NB: *specialist use only* – strongly consider getting senior help before giving.

☠ Toxic if extravasation when given iv (⇒ tissue necrosis)☠.

SODIUM VALPROATE see Valproate; antiepileptic.

SOTALOL

β-Blocker (non-selective); class II (+III) antiarrhythmic.

Use: Px of SVT (esp of paroxysmal AF), **Rx of VT**(if life-threatening/ symptomatic, esp non-sustained or spontaneous sustained dt IHD or cardiomyopathy).

CI: as propranolol, plus ↑QT syndromes, torsades de pointes, **R** (if severe, otherwise caution).

Caution: as propranolol, plus electrolyte Δs (⇒ ↑risk of arrhythmias, esp if ↓K^+/↓ Mg^{2+}; ∴ beware if severe diarrhoea).

SE: as propranolol, plus arrhythmias (can ⇒ ↑QT ± **torsadesde pointes***, esp in females).

Interactions: as propranolol (NB: ☠ *Verapamil and diltiazem* ⇒*risk of ↓HR and HB*☠) plus disopyramides, quinidine, procainamide, amiodarone, moxifloxacin, mizolastine, dolasetron, ivabradine, TCAs and antipsychotics ⇒ ↑**risk arrhythmias***.

Dose: 40–160 mg bd po (↑if life-threatening to max 640 mg/day); 20–120 mg iv over 10 min (repeat 6 - hrly if necessary). **NB: ↓dose if RF.**

Give under specialist supervision and with ECG monitoring.

SPIRIVA see Tiotropium; new inhaled muscarinic antagonist.
▼ Respimat (non Handihaler).

SPIRONOLACTONE

K^+-sparing diuretic: aldosterone antagonist at distal tubule (also potentiates loop and thiazidediuretics).

Use: ascites (esp 2° to cirrhosis or malignancy), oedema, HF (adjunct to ACE-i and/or another diuretic), nephrotic syndrome, 1° aldosteronism.

CI: ↑K^+, ↓Na^+, Addison's, **P/B**.

Caution: porphyria, **L/R/E**.

SE: ↑K⁺, **gynaecomastia**, GI upset (inc N&V), impotence, ↓BP,↑Na⁺, rash, confusion, headache, hepatotoxicity, blood disorders.

Monitor: U&E.

Interactions: ↑s digoxin and lithium levels. ↑s risk of RF with NSAIDs (which also antagonise its diuretic fx).

Dose: 100–400 mg/day po (25 mg od if for HF).

> ☠Beware if on other drugs that ↑K⁺, e.g. amiloride, triamterene, ACE-i, angiotensin II antagonists and ciclosporin. Do not give with oral K⁺ supplements inc dietary salt substitutes☠.

STEMETIL see Prochlorperazine; DA antagonist antiemetic.

STREPTOKINASE

Thrombolytic agent: ↑s plasminogen conversion to plasmin ⇒↑fibrin breakdown.

Use: AMI, TE of arteries (inc PE, central retinal artery) or veins (DVT, central retinal vein).

CI/Caution/SE: see p. 215.

Dose: AMI: 1.5 million units ivi over 60 min; **other indications:** 250000 units ivi over 30 min, then 100000 units ivi every hour for up to 12–72 h (see SPC).

STREPTOMYCIN

Aminoglycoside antibiotic.

Use: TB (if isoniazid resistance established before Rx); see p. 175.

CI/Caution/SE/Interactions: see Gentamicin.

STRONTIUM RANELATE/PROTELOS

↑s bone formation and ↓s bone resorption.

Use: postmenopausal osteoporosis^NICE if bisphosphonates CI/not tolerated & aged >75 with previous fracture.

CI: phenylketonuria (contains aspartame), **P/B**.

Caution: ↑risk of VTE, Δs urinary and plasma Ca²⁺ measurements. **R** (avoid if severe).

SE: severe allergic reactions* GI upset.

Warn: to report any skin rash* and immediately stop drug.

Interactions: absorption ↓ by concomitant ingestion of Ca^{2+} (e.g. milk) and Mg^{2+}. ↓s absorption of quinolones and tetracycline.

Dose: 2 g (1 sachet in water) po od at bedtime[SPC/BNF]. *Avoid food/ milk 2 h before and after taking.*

> 💀Rash* can be early DRESS syndrome: Drug Rash, Eosinophilia and Systemic Symptoms (e.g. fever); lymphadenopathy and ↑WCC also seen early. Can ⇒ LF, RF or respiratory failure ± death💀.

SULFASALAZINE

Aminosalicylate: combination of the immune modulator 5 - aminosalicylic acid (5-ASA) and the antibacterial sulfapyridine (a sulphonamide).

Use: rheumatoid arthritis[1]. Also UC[2] (inc maintenance of remission) and active Crohn's disease[2], but not 1st-line, as newer drugs (e.g. mesalazine) have ↓sulphonamide SEs; still used if well-controlled with this drug and with no SEs or if joint manifestations.

CI: sulphonamide or salicylate hypersensitivity, **R** (caution if mild).

Caution: slow acetylators, Hx of any allergy, porphyria, G6PD deficiency, **L/P** (give only under specialist care)/**B**.

SE: GI upset (esp ↓appetite/Wt), **hepatotoxicity**, **blood disorders**, **hypersensitivity** (inc severe skin reactions like Stevens–Johnson syndrome), seizures, lupus.

Monitor: LFTs, U&Es, FBC.

Dose: 500 mg/day ↑ing to max 3 g/day[1]; 1–2 g qds po for acute attacks[2], ↓ing to maintenance of 500 mg qds – can also give 0.5–1.0 g pr bd after motion (as supps) ± po Rx.

SUMATRIPTAN/IMIGRAN

$5HT_{1B/1D}$ agonist.

Use: migraine (acute). Also cluster headache (sc route only).

CI: IHD, coronary vasospasm (inc Prinzmetal's), PVD, HTN (moderate, severe or uncontrolled). Hx of MI, CVA or TIA.

Caution: predisposition to IHD (e.g. cardiac disease), **L/H/P/B/E**.

SE: sensory Δs (tingling, heat, pressure/tightness), dizziness, flushing, fatigue, N&V, seizures, visual Δs and drowsiness.

Interactions: ↑risk of CNS toxicity with SSRIs, MAOIs, moclobemide and St John's wort. ↑risk of vasospasm with ergotamine and methysergide.

Dose: 50 mg po (can repeat after ≥2 h if responded then recurs and can ↑doses, **if no LF**, to 100 mg if required). Max 300 mg/24 h. Available sc or intranasally[BNF/SPC].

NB: frequent use may ⇒ medication overuse headache.

SYMBICORT Combination asthma inhaler: each puff contains x microgram budesonide (steroid) + y microgram formoterol (long-acting β_2 agonist) in the following 'x/y' strengths; '100/6', '200/6' and '400/12'.

SYNACTHEN SYNthetic ACTH (adreno cortico trophic hormone), also called tetracosactide.

Use: Dx of Addison's disease: in 'short' syncathen test will find ↓plasma cortisol 0, 30 and 60 min after 250 microgram iv/im dose.

CI: allergic disorders (esp asthma). NB: can ⇒ anaphylaxis.

TACROLIMUS (= FK 506)

Immunosuppressant (calcineurin inhibitor): ↓s IL-2-mediated LØ proliferation.

Use: Px of transplant rejection (esp renal). Also used topically as 0.1% or 0.03% ointment in moderate-severe atopic eczema unresponsive to conventional therapy (specialist use).

CI: macrolide hypersensitivity, immunodeficiency, **P** (exclude before starting), **B**.

Caution/SE: as ciclosporin, but ⇒ ↑neuro-/nephro-toxicity (although ⇒ ↓hypertrichosis/hirsutism); also **diabetogenic** and rarely ⇒cardiomyopathy (monitor ECG for hypertrophic Δs).

Interactions: metab by **P450** ∴ many, but most importantly: ↑s levels of ☙ciclosporin☙. Levels ↑ by clari-/ery-/teli-thromycin, quinu-/dalfo-pristin, chloramphenicol, antifungals, ataza-/rito-/nelfi-/

saqui-navir, nifedipine, diltiazem and grapefruit juice. Levels ↓ by rifampicin, phenobarbital, phenytoin and St John's wort. Nephrotoxicity↑ by NSAIDs, aminoglycosides and amphotericin. Avoid with other drugs that ↑K+.

Dose: specialist use[SPC/BNF]. ▼ Modigraf (not other brands) **NB: may require ↓dose if LF.**

> Interactions important: ↑levels ⇒ toxicity; ↓levels may ⇒ rejection. Available in immediate release & modified release preparations with different dosing; Prograf, Adoport & Modigraf (bd) and Advagraf (MR od preparation) ∴ mustn't confuse .

TADALAFIL/CIALIS/ADCIRCA (▼)

Phosphodiesterase type-5 inhibitor; see Sildenafil.

CI/Use/Caution/SE/Interactions: as sildenafil plus CI in moderate HF and uncontrolled HTN/arrhythmias.

Dose (*for erectile dysfunction*): initially 10 mg ≥30 min before sexual activity, adjusting to response (1 dose per 24 h, max 20 mg per dose, unless RF or LF when max 10 mg).

TAMOXIFEN

Oestrogen receptor antagonist.

Use: oestrogen receptor-positive Ca breast[1] (as adjuvant Rx: ⇒ ↑survival, delays metastasis), anovulatory infertility[2].

CI: P** (exclude pregnancy before starting Rx).

Caution: ↑risk of TE* (if taking cytotoxics), porphyria, B.

SE: hot flushes, GI upset, menstrual/endometrial Δs (inc Ca: if Δ vaginal bleeding/discharge or pelvic pain/pressure ⇒ urgent Ix). Also fluid retention, exac of bony metastases pain. Many other gynaecological/blood/skin/metabolic Δs (esp lipids, LFTs).

Warn: of symptoms of endometrial cancer and TE* (and to report calf pain/sudden SOB). If appropriate, advise non-hormonal contraception**.

Interactions: W + .

Dose: 20 mg od po[1]; for anovulatory infertility[2] see SPC/BNF.

TAMSULOSIN/FLOMAXTRA XL

α-Blocker ⇒ internal urethral sphincter relaxation (∴ ⇒ ↑bladder outflow) and systemic vasodilation.
Use: BPH.
CI/Caution/SE/Interactions: as doxazosin plus **L** (if severe).
Dose: 400 microgram mane (after food).

TAZOCIN Combination of piperacillin (antipseudomonal penicillin) + tazobactam (β-lactamase inhibitor).
Use: severe infections/sepsis (mostly in ITU setting or if resistant to other antibiotics).
CI/Caution/SE/Interactions: as benzylpenicillin.
Dose: 2.25–4.5 g tds/qds iv. NB: ↓to bd/tds if RF.

TEGRETOL see Carbamazepine; antiepileptic.

TEICOPLANIN

Glycopeptide antibiotic.
Use: serious Gram-positive infections (mostly reserved for MRSA).
Caution: vancomycin sensitivity, R/P/B/E.
SE: GI upset, hypersensitivity/skin reactions, blood disorders, nephrotoxicity, ototoxicity (but less than vancomycin), ΔLFTs, local reactions at injection site.
Monitor: U&Es, LFTs, FBC, auditory function (esp if chronic Rx or on other oto-/nephro-toxic drugs, e.g. gentamicin, amphotericin B, ciclosporin, cisplatin and furosemide). Drug levels may be monitored in some situations – consult local guidelines/experts.
Dose: single loading dose of 400 mg im/iv, then ↓ to 200 mg od 24 h later (if severe infection continue at 400 mg 12-hrly for 2 more doses before changing to 200 mg od; if life-threatening continue at 400 mg od). NB: ↑dose if weight ≥85 kg, severe burns or endocarditis and ↓dose if RF; see SPC/BNF.

▼ TELMISARTAN/MICARDIS

Angiotensin II antagonist; see Losartan.

Use: HTN; *for advice on stepped HTN Mx see p. 182.*
CI: biliary obstruction, **L** (if severe, otherwise caution), **P/B**.
Caution/SE/Interactions: as Losartan, plus ↑s digoxin levels.
Dose: 20–80 mg od (usually 40 mg od). NB: ↓dose if LF or RF.

TEMAZEPAM

Benzodiazepine, short-acting.
Use: insomnia.
CI/Caution/SE/Interactions: see Diazepam.
Dose: 10 mg nocte (can ↑dose if tolerant to benzodiazepines, but beware respiratory depression). *Dependency common*: max 4-wk Rx.
NB: ↓dose if LF, severe RF or elderly.

TENECTEPLASE (= TNK-tPA)/METALYSE

Recombinant thrombolytic; advantageous as given as single bolus.
Use: Acute myocardial infarction.
CI/Caution/SE: see p. 215, plus **B**.
Dose: iv bolus over 10 sec according to weight: ≥ 90 kg, 50 mg; 80–89 kg, 45 mg; 70–79 kg, 40 mg; 60–69 kg, 35 mg; < 60 kg, 30 mg.

Concurrent unfractionated iv heparin or enoxaparin is needed for 24–48 h; see p. 215.

TERAZOSIN/HYTRIN

α-Blocker ⇒ internal urethral sphincter relaxation (∴ ⇒ ↑bladder outflow) and systemic vasodilation.
Use: BPH[1] (and rarely HTN[2]).
Caution: Hx of micturition syncope or postural ↓BP, **P/B/E**.
SE/Interactions: see Doxazosin. '1st-dose collapse' common.
Dose: initially 1 mg nocte, ↑ing as necessary to max 10 mg/day[1] (or 20 mg/day[2]).

TERBINAFINE/LAMISIL

Antifungal: oral[1,2] or topical cream[3].
Use: ringworm[1] (*Tinea* spp), dermatophyte nail infections[2], fungal skin infections[3]. NB: ineffective in yeast infections.

Caution: psoriasis (may worsen), autoimmune disease (risk of lupus-like syndrome), **L/R** (neither apply if giving topically), **P/B**.
SE: headache, GI upset, mild rash, joint/muscle pains. Rarely neuro-Ψ disturbances, blood disorders, hepatic dysfunction, serious skin reactions (stop drug if progressive rash).
Dose: 250 mg od po for 2–6 wks[1] or 6 wks–3 months[2]; 1–2 topical applications/day for 1–2 wks[3].

TERBUTALINE/BRICANYL

Inhaled β_2 agonist similar to salbutamol.
Dose: 250–500 microgram od–qds inh (powder or aerosol); 5–10 mg up to qds neb. Can also give po/sc/im/iv[SPC/BNF].

TETRACYCLINE

Tetracycline broad-spectrum antibiotic: inhibits ribosomal (30S subunit) protein synthesis.
Use: acne vulgaris[1] (or rosacea), genital/tropical infections (NB: doxycycline often preferred).
CI: age < 12 years (**stains/deforms teeth**), acute porphyria, **R/P/B**.
Caution: may worsen MG or SLE, **L**.
SE: GI upset (rarely AAC), oesophageal irritation, headache, dysphagia. Rarely hepatotoxicity, blood disorders, photosensitivity, hypersensitivity, visual Δs (rarely 2° to BIH; stop drug if suspected).
Interactions: ↓absorption with milk (do not drink 1 h before or 2 h after drug), antacids and Fe/Al/Ca/Mg/Zn salts. ↓s fx of OCP (small risk). ↑risk of BIH with retinoids. Mild **W +** .
Dose: 500 mg bd po[1], otherwise 250–500 mg tds/qds po. NB: **max 1 g/24 h in LF.**

NB: take > 30 min before food.

THEOPHYLLINE

Methylxanthine bronchodilator. *Theories of action*: (1) ↑s intracellular cAMP; (2) adenosine antagonist; (3) ↓s diaphragm fatigue. NB: additive fx with β_2 agonists (but with ↑risk of SEs, esp ↓K^+).

Use: severe asthma/COPD: acute (iv as aminophylline; see p. 247) or chronic (po; see p. 186 for BTS asthma guidelines).

CI: hypersensitivity to any 'xanthine' (e.g. aminophylline/theophylline), acute porphyria.

Caution: cardiac disease (risk of arrhythmias*), epilepsy, $\uparrow T_4$, PU, HTN, fever, porphyria, acute febrile illness, glaucoma, DM, L/P/B/E.

SE: (tachy)**arrhythmias***, seizures (esp if given rapidly iv), **GI upset** (esp **nausea**), CNS stimulation (restlessness, insomnia), headache, $\downarrow K^+$.

Monitor: K^+, serum levels (4–6 h post dose) as narrow therapeutic window (10–20 mg/l = 55–110 micromol/l) but toxic fx can occur even in this range.

Interactions: metab by **P450** ($\Rightarrow$ very variable $t_{1/2}$): **levels $\uparrow$d** in HF/LF*/viral infections/elderly, and if taking **fluvoxamine**/cimetidine/ciprofloxacin/norfloxacin/macrolides (ery-/clari-thromycin)/propranolol/'flu vaccines/fluconazole/ketoconazole/OCP/Ca^{2+} channel blockers. **Levels $\downarrow$d in** smokers/chronic alcohol abuse, and if taking phenytoin/carbamazepine/phenobarbital/rifampicin/ritonavir/St John's wort. $\uparrow$risk of convulsions with quinolones.

Dose: MR preparations preferred ($\downarrow$SEs) and doses vary with brand[SPC/BNF]; range 200–500 mg bd. *Available iv as aminophylline.* NB: $\downarrow$**dose if LF***. Note: dose adjustment may be necessary if smoking started or stopped during chronic treatment.

THIAMINE (= vitamin B1).

Use: replacement for nutritional deficiencies (esp in alcoholism).

Dose: 100 mg bd/tds po in severe deficiency (25 mg od if mild/chronic).

For iv preparations, see Pabrinex and p. 195 for Mx of acute alcohol withdrawal.

THYROXINE (= LEVOTHYROXINE).

Synthetic T_4 (NB: thyroxine often now called 'levothyroxine').

Use: $\downarrow T_4$ Rx (for maintenance); **NB:** acutely, e.g. myxoedema coma, liothyronine (T_3) often needed – see p. 257.

CI: ↑T_4.

Caution: panhypopituitarism/other predisposition to adrenal insufficiency (*corticosteroids needed 1st*), chronic ↓T_4, cardiovascular disorders (esp HTN/IHD; can worsen)*, DI, DM**, **P/B/E**.

SE: features of ↑T_4 (should be minimal unless xs Rx): D&V, tremors, restlessness, headache, flushing, sweating, heat intolerance, angina, arrhythmias, palpitations, ↑HR, muscle cramps/weakness, ↓Wt. Also osteoporosis (esp if xs dose given; use min dose necessary).

Interactions: can Δ digoxin and antidiabetic** requirements, ↑fx of TCAs and ↓levels of propranolol. **W** + .

Monitor: baseline ECG to help distinguish Δs due to ischaemia or ↓T_4.

Dose: 25–200 microgram mane (titrate up slowly, esp if > 50 yrs old/↓↓T_4/HTN/IHD*).

TIMOLOL EYE DROPS/TIMOPTOL

β-Blocker eye drops; ↓aqueous humour production.

Use: glaucoma (2nd line), ocular HTN (1st line); not useful if on systemic β-blocker.

CI: asthma, ↓HR, HB, **H** (if uncontrolled).

Caution/SE/Interactions: as propranolol* plus can ⇒ local irritation.

Dose: 1 drop bd (0.25% or 0.5%). Also available in long-acting od preparations TIMOPTOL LA (0.25 and 0.5%) and NYOGEL (0.1%). Timolol 0.5% also available in combination with other classes of glaucoma medications; carbonic anhydrase inhibitors (dorzolamide Cosopt, brinzolamide ▼ Azarga), PG analogues (latanoprost Xalacom, travoprost Duotrav, bimatoprost Ganfort) α-agonists (brimonidine Combigan).

☠ Systemic absorption possible despite topical application* ☠ .

TINZAPARIN/INNOHEP

Low-molecular-weight heparin (LMWH).

Use: DVT/PE Rx[1] and Px[2] (inc pre-operative). Not licensed for MI/unstable angina (unlike other LMWHs).

CI/Caution/SE/Monitor/Interactions: as heparin, plus CI if breast feeding (**B**) and caution in asthma ($\Rightarrow$ $\uparrow$hypersensitivity reactions).
Dose: (all sc) 175 units/kg od[1]; 50 units/kg or 4500 units od[2] (3500 units od if low risk).

Consider monitoring anti-Xa (3–4 h post dose) $\pm$ dose adjustment if RF (i.e. creatinine >150), severe LF, pregnancy, Wt >100 kg or <45 kg; see p. 212.

TIOTROPIUM/SPIRIVA

Long-acting in h muscarinic antagonist for COPD/asthma; similar to ipratropium, but only for chronic use and caution in RF.
SE: dry mouth, urinary retention, glaucoma.
Dose: 18 microgram dry powder inhaler or 5 microgram by soft mist inhaler od inh.

TIROFIBAN/AGGRASTAT

Antiplatelet agent: glycoprotein IIb/IIIa receptor inhibitor – stops binding of fibrinogen and inhibits platelet aggregation.
Use: Px of MI in unstable angina/NSTEMI (*if last episode of chest pain w/in 12 h*), esp if high risk and awaiting PCI[NICE] (see p. 240).
CI: abnormal bleeding or CVA w/in 30 days, haemorrhagic diathesis, Hx of haemorrhagic CVA, intracranial disease (neoplasm/aneurysm/AVM), severe HTN, $\downarrow$Pt, $\uparrow$INR/PT, **B**.
Caution: $\uparrow$risk of bleeding (e.g. drugs, recent bleeding/trauma/procedures; see[SPC/BNF]), **L** (avoid if severe), **H** (if severe), **R/P**.
SE: bleeding, nausea, fever, $\downarrow$Pt (reversible).
Monitor: FBC (baseline, 2–6 h after giving, then at least daily).
Dose: 400 *nanograms*/kg/min for 30 min, then 100 *nanograms*/kg/min for $\geq$48 h (continue for 12–24 h post-PCI), for max of 108 h. Needs concurrent heparin. NB: $\downarrow$**dose if RF**.

Specialist use only: get senior advice or contact on-call cardiology.

TOLBUTAMIDE

Oral antidiabetic (short-acting sulphonylurea).

Use/CI/Caution/SE/Interactions: as gliclazide. Can also ⇒ headache and tinnitus. fx ↑ by azapropazone.
Dose: 0.5–2.0 g daily in divided doses, with food. NB: ↓dose if RF or LF.

TOLTERODINE/DETRUSITOL

Antimuscarinic, antispasmodic.
Use: detrusor instability; urinary incontinence/frequency/urgency.
CI/Caution/SE: as oxybutynin (SEs mostly antimuscarinic fx; see p. 233) plus caution if Hx of, or taking drugs that, ↑QTc, **P/B**.
Interactions: ↑risk of ventricular arrhythmias with amiodarone, disopyramide, flecainide and sotalol.
Dose: 1–2 mg bd po. NB: ↓dose if RF or LF. (MR preparation available as 4 mg od po; not suitable if RF or LF.)

tPA (= tissue-type plasminogen activator) see Alteplase.

TRAMADOL

Opioid. Also ↓s pain by ↑ing 5HT/noradrenergic transmission.
Use: moderate/severe pain (esp musculoskeletal).
CI/Caution: as codeine, but also CI in uncontrolled epilepsy, **P/B**. Not suitable as substitute in opioid-dependent patients.
SE: as morphine, but ↓respiratory depression, ↓constipation, ↓addiction. ↑confusion (esp in elderly) compared to codeine.
Interactions: as codeine; also ↑risk convulsions with SSRIs/TCAs/antipsychotics, ↑risk serotonin syndrome with SSRIs. Carbamazepine and ondansetron ↓ its fx. **W +**.
Dose: 50–100 mg up to 4-hrly po/im/iv, max 400 mg/day. Post-op: initially 100 mg im/iv, then 50 mg every 10–20 min prn (max total dose of 250 mg in 1st hr), then 50–100 mg 4–6-hrly (max 600 mg/day). NB: ↓dose if RF, LF or elderly.

TRANDOLAPRIL/GOPTEN

ACE-i for HTN (*for advice on stepped HTN Mx see p. 182*), HF and LVF post-MI.
CI/Caution/SE/Monitor/Interactions: see Captopril.

Dose: initially 0.5 mg od, ↑ing at intervals of 2–4 wks if required to max 4 mg od (max 2 mg if RF). ↓doses if given with diuretic. If for LVF post-MI, start ≥3 days after MI.

TRANEXAMIC ACID

Antifibrinolytic: inhibits activation of plasminogen to plasmin.
Use: bleeding: acute bleeds[1] (esp 2° to anticoagulants, thrombolytic/anti-Pt agents, epistaxis, haemophilia), menorrhagia[2], hereditary angioedema[3].
CI: TE disease, **R** (if severe, otherwise caution).
Caution: gross haematuria (can clot and obstruct ureters), DIC, **P**.
SE: GI upset, colour vision Δs (stop drug), TE.
Dose: 15–25 mg/kg bd/tds po (if severe, 0.5–1 g tds iv)[1]; 1 g tds po for 4 days (max 4 g/day)[2]; 1–1.5 g bd/tds po[3]. **NB:** ↓**dose if RF.**

TRAVOPROST EYE DROPS/TRAVATAN

Topical PG analogue for glaucoma; see Latanoprost.
Use/CI/Caution/SE: see Latanoprost.
Dose: 1 drop od.

TRIAMTERENE

K^+-sparing diuretic (weak); see Amiloride.
Use/CI/Caution/SE: as amiloride, but ⇒ less ↓BP ∴ not used for HTN (unless used with other drugs), plus **L** (avoid if severe).
Warn: urine may go blue.
Interactions: ↑s lithium, phenobarbital and amantadine levels. NSAIDs ↑risk of RF and ↑K^+.
Dose: almost exclusively used with stronger K^+-wasting diuretics in combination preparations (e.g. co-triamterzide). For use alone, initially give 150–250 mg daily, ↓ing to alternate days after 1wk.

☠ Beware if on other drugs that ↑K^+, e.g. amiloride, spironolactone, ACE-i, angiotensin II antagonists and ciclosporin. Do not give with oral K^+ tablets or dietary salt substitutes ☠.

TRI-IODOTHYRONINE

See Liothyronine; synthetic T$_3$ mostly used in myxoedema coma.

TRIMETHOPRIM

Antifolate antibiotic: inhibits dihydrofolate reductase.
Use: UTIs (rarely other infections).
CI: blood disorders (esp megaloblastic ↓Hb).
Caution: ↓folate (or predisposition to), porphyria, R/P/B/E.
SE: see Co-trimoxazole (Septrin), but much less frequent and severe
(esp BM suppression, skin reactions). Also **GI upset**, rash, rarely other
hypersensitivity.
Warn: those on long-term Rx to look for signs of blood disorder and
to report fever, sore throat, rash, mouth ulcers, bruising or bleeding.
Interactions: ↑s phenytoin levels. ↑s risk of arrhythmias with
amiodarone, antifolate fx with pyrimethamine and toxicity with
ciclosporin, azathioprine, mercaptopurine and methotrexate. **W +**.
Dose: 200 mg bd po (100 mg nocte for chronic infections or as Px if
at risk; NB: risk of ↓folate if long-term Rx). **NB: ↓dose if RF**.

TROPICAMIDE EYE DROPS

Antimuscarinic: mydriatic (lasts approx 4 hrs), weak cycloplegic.
Use: dilated retinal examination. See also 'Dilating eye drops'.
CI: untreated acute angle closure glaucoma.
Caution: ↑IOP* (inc predisposition to), inflamed eye (↑risk of
systemic absorption).
SE: transient stinging & blurred vision & ↓accommodation. Rarely
precipitation of acute angle closure glaucoma (↑risk if >60 yrs, long
sighted, family history).
Warn: unable to drive until can read car number plate at 20 metres
(approx 4 hrs).
Dose: 1 drop 1.0% solution 15–20 min before examination. 0.5% in
children <1 yr old. NB: Rare cause of acute angle closure glaucoma*
(esp if >60 yrs or hypermetropic).

TURBOHALER Inh delivery device for asthma drugs.

(SODIUM) VALPROATE

Antiepileptic and mood stabiliser: potentiates and ↑s GABA levels.

Use: epilepsy[1], mania (and off-licence for other Ψ disorders).

CI: acute porphyria, personal or family Hx of severe liver dysfunction, **L** (inc active liver disease).

Caution: SLE, ↑bleeding risk*, **R**, **P** (⇒ neural-tube/craniofacial dfx, Px folate), **B**.

SE: sedation, cerebellar fx (see p. 236; esp tremor, ataxia), **headache**, **GI upset**, ↑Wt, SOA, alopecia, skin reactions, ↓cognitive/motor function, Ψ disorders, encephalopathy (2° to ↑NH). Rarely but seriously **hepatotoxicity**, **blood disorders** (esp ↓Pt*), **pancreatitis** (mostly in 1st 6 months of Rx).

Warn: of clinical features of pancreatitis and liver/blood disorders. Inform women of childbearing age of teratogenicity/need for contraception.

Monitor: LFTs, FBC ± serum levels *pre-dose* (therapeutic range 50–100 mg/l; useful for checking compliance but ↓use for efficacy).

Interactions: fx ↓d by antimalarials (esp mefloquine), antidepressants (inc St John's wort), antipsychotics and some antiepileptics[SPC/BNF]. Levels ↑by cimetidine & carbopenems. ↑s fx of aspirin and primidone. ↑risk of ↓NØ with olanzapine. Mild **W** + .

Dose: initially 300 mg bd, ↑ing to max of 2.5 g/day[1]. NB: ↓dose if RF.

Can give false-positive urine dipstick for ketones.

▼ VALSARTAN/DIOVAN

Angiotensin II antagonist; see Losartan.

Use: HTN[1] (*for advice on stepped HTN Mx see p. 182*), MI with LV failure/dysfunction[2], heart failure[3].

CI: biliary obstruction, cirrhosis, **L** (if severe)/**P/B**.

Caution/SE/Interactions: see Losartan (inc warning r/e drugs that ↑K+).

Dose: initially 80 mg od[1] (NB: give 40 mg if ≥75 yrs old, LF, RF or ↓intravascular volume) or 20 mg bd[2,3], ↑ing if necessary to max 320 mg od[1]/160 mg bd[2] or 40 mg bd[3].

VANCOMYCIN

Glycopeptide antibiotic. Poor po absorption (unless bowel inflammation*), but still effective against C. *difficile*** as acts 'topically' in GI tract.

Use: serious Gram-positive infections[1] (inc endocarditis Px and systemic MRSA), AAC[2] (give po)**.

Caution: Hx of deafness, IBD* (only if given po), avoid rapid infusions (risk of anaphylaxis), R/P/B/E.

SE: nephrotoxicity, ototoxicity (stop if tinnitus develops), **blood disorders, rash, hypersensitivity** (inc anaphylaxis, severe skin reactions), nausea, fever, phlebitis/irritation at injection site.

Monitor: serum levels: keep predose trough levels 10–15 mg/l; start monitoring after 3rd dose (1st dose if RF); NB: higher trough recommended in osteomyelitis, endocarditis. Also monitor U&Es, FBC, urinalysis (and auditory function if elderly/RF).

Interactions: ↑nephrotoxicity with ciclosporin. ↑ototoxicity with loop diuretics. ↑s fx of suxamethonium.

Dose: 1–1.5 g bd ivi over 100 min[1]; 125 mg qds po[2]. **NB: ↓dose if RF or elderly.**

NB: if ivi given too quickly ⇒ ↑risk of anaphylactoid reactions (e.g. ↓BP, respiratory symptoms, skin reactions).

VARDENAFIL/LEVITRA

Phosphodiesterase type-5 inhibitor; see Sildenafil.

Use/CI/Caution/SE/Interactions: as sildenafil plus CI in hereditary degenerative retinal disorders, caution if susceptible to (or taking drugs that) ↑QTc, and levels ↑by grapefruit juice.

Dose: initially 10 mg approx 25–60 min before sexual activity, adjusting to response (1 dose per 24 h, max 20 mg per dose).
NB: halve dose if LF, RF, elderly or taking α-blocker.

VENLAFAXINE/EFEXOR

Serotonin and Noradrenaline Reuptake Inhibitor (SNRI): antidepressant with ↓sedative/antimuscarinic fx cf TCAs. ↑danger in OD/heart disease than other antidepressants; see p. 197.

Use: depression[1], generalised anxiety disorder.

CI: very high risk of serious cardiac ventricular arrhythmia (e.g. significant LV dysfunction, NYHA class III/IV), uncontrolled HTN, **P**.

Caution: Hx of mania, seizures or glaucoma, **L/R** (avoid if either severe) **H/B**.

SE: GI upset, ↑BP (dose-related; monitor BP if dose >200 mg/day), **withdrawal fx** (see p. 235; common even if dose only a few hours late), **rash** (consider stopping drug, as can be 1st sign of severe reaction*), insomnia/agitation, dry mouth, sexual dysfunction, ↑weight, drowsiness, dizziness, SIADH and ↑QTc.

Warn: report rashes* and can ↓driving/skilled task ability. Don't stop suddenly.

Monitor: BP if heart disease ± ECG.

Interactions: ☠ *Never give with, or ≤2 wks after, MAOIs* ☠. ↑s risk of bleeding with aspirin/NSAIDs and CNS toxicity with selegiline/sibutramine. Avoid artemether/lumefantrine. ↑s levels of clozapine. Mild **W+**.

Dose: 37.5–187.5 mg bd po[1]; start low and ↑dose if required. Efexor XL MR od preparation available (max 225 mg od). *NB: halve dose if moderate LF (PT 14–18 s) or RF (GFR 10–30 ml/min).*

VENTOLIN see Salbutamol; β-agonist bronchodilator.

VERAPAMIL

Ca^{2+} channel blocker (rate-limiting type): fx on heart (⇒ ↓HR, ↓contractility*) > vasculature (dilates peripheral/coronary arteries); i.e. reverse of the dihydropyridine type (e.g. nifedipine). Only Ca^{2+} channel blocker with useful antiarrhythmic properties (class IV).

Use: HTN[1] *(for advice on stepped HTN Mx see p. 182)*, angina[2], arrhythmias (SVTs, esp instead of adenosine if asthma)[3].

CI: ↓BP, ↓HR (<50 bpm), 2nd-/3rd-degree HB, ↓LV function, SAN block, SSS, AF or atrial flutter 2° to WPW, acute porphyria. **H*** (inc Hx of).

Caution: AMI, 1st degree HB, **L/P/B**.

SE: constipation (rarely other GI upset), HF, ↓BP (dose-dependent), HB, headache, dizziness, fatigue, ankle oedema, hypersensitivity, skin reactions.

Interactions: ↑risk of AV block and HF with ☠ β-blockers ☠ disopyramide, flecainide and amiodarone. ↑s hypotensive fx of antihypertensives (esp α-blockers) and anaesthetics. ↑s levels/fx of digoxin, theophyllines, carbamazepine, quinidine, ivabradine and ciclosporin. Levels/fx ↓by rifampicin, barbiturates and primidone. ↑risk of myopathy with simvastatin. Sirolimus ↑s levels of both drugs. Levels may be ↑by clari-/ery-thromycin and ritonavir. Risk of VF with ☠ iv dantrolene ☠.

Warn: fx ↑d by grapefruit juice (avoid).

Dose: 80–160 mg tds po[1]; 80–120 mg tds po[2]; 40–120 mg tds po[3]; 5–10 mg iv (over 2 min (3 min in elderly) with ECG monitoring), followed by additional 5 mg iv if necessary after 5–10 min[3]. MR (od/bd) preparations available[BNF]. **NB:** ↓oral dose in LF.

VIAGRA see Sildenafil; phosphodiesterase inhibitor.

VITAMIN K see Phytomenadione.

VOLTAROL see Diclofenac; moderate-strength NSAID.

WARFARIN

Oral anticoagulant: blocks synthesis of vitamin-K-dependent factors (II, VII, IX, X) and proteins C and S.

Use: Rx/Px of TE; see p. 207.

CI: severe HTN, PU, bacterial endocarditis, **P**.

Caution: recent surgery, **L/R** (avoid if creatinine clearance < 10 ml/min)/**B**.

SE: **haemorrhage**, rash, fever, diarrhoea. Rarely other GI upset, 'purple-toe syndrome', skin necrosis, hepatotoxicity, hypersensitivity.

Warn: fx are ↑d by alcohol and cranberry juice (avoid).

Dose: see p. 207.

> ☠ NB: **W+** and **W–** denote significant interactions throughout this book: take particular care with antibiotics and drugs that affect cytochrome **P450** (see p. 237) ☠.

XALATAN see ▼ Latanoprost; topical PG analogue for glaucoma.

ZALEPLON

'Non-benzodiazepine' hypnotic; see Zopiclone.
Use/CI/Caution/SE/Interactions: see Zopiclone.
Dose: 10 mg nocte (5 mg if elderly). NB: halve dose if LF (avoid if severe), severe RF or elderly.

ZANTAC see Ranitidine; H antagonist.

ZESTRIL see Lisinopril; ACE-i.

ZIDOVUDINE (AZT)

Antiviral (nucleoside analogue): reverse-transcriptase inhibitor.
Use: HIV Rx (and Px, esp of vertical transmission).
CI: severe $\downarrow$NØ or $\downarrow$Hb (caution if other blood disorders), acute porphyria, **B**.
Caution: $\downarrow$B12, $\uparrow$risk of lactic acidosis, **L/R/P/E**.
SE: blood disorders (esp $\downarrow$Hb or $\downarrow$WCC), **GI upset, headache, fever**, taste Δs, sleep disorders. Rarely hepatic/pancreatic dysfunction, myopathy, seizures, other neurological/Ψ disorders.
Interactions: levels $\uparrow$ by fluconazole. fx $\downarrow$ by ritonavir. $\uparrow$myelosuppression with ganciclovir. $\uparrow$risk of $\downarrow$Hb with ribavirin. $\downarrow$s fx of stavudine and tipranavir.
Dose: see SPC/BNF.

ZIRTEK see Cetirizine; non-sedating antihistamine for allergies.

ZOLEDRONIC ACID/ZOMETA

Bisphosphonate: $\downarrow$s osteoclastic bone resorption.
Use: Px of bone damage[1] in advanced bone malignancy, damage or Rx of $\uparrow$Ca^{2+} in malignancy[2], Rx of Paget's disease of bone[3], Rx of osteoporosis (postmenopausal or in men)[4].
CI: P/B.
Caution: cardiac disease, dehydration*, $\downarrow$Ca^{2+}/PO$_4^{2-}$/Mg^{2+}. **L** (if severe)/**R/H**.
SE: 'flu-like syndrome, fever, bone pain, fatigue, N&V. Also arthr-/my-algia, $\downarrow$Ca^{2+}/PO$_4^{2-}$/Mg^{2+}, pruritus/rash, headache,

conjunctivitis, RF, hypersensitivity, blood disorders (esp ↓Hb) and **osteonecrosis** (esp of jaw; consider dental examination or preventive Rx before starting drug).

Monitor: Ca^{2+}, PO_4^{2-}, Mg^{2+}, U&E. Ensure patient adequately hydrated predose* and advise good dental hygiene.

Dose: 4 mg ivi every 3–4 weeks[1]; 4 mg ivi as single dose[2]. Also available as once yearly preparation (▼ Aclasta) 5 mg ivi over ≥ 15 mins[3,4]. NB: ↓**dose in RF.**

ZOLMITRIPTAN/ZOMIG

$5HT_{1B/1D}$ agonist for acute migraine.

Use/CI/Caution/SE/Interactions: as sumatriptan plus CI in WPW or arrhythmias assoc with accessory cardiac conduction p'way.

Dose: 2.5 mg po (can repeat after ≥ 2 h if responded then recurs and can ↑doses to 5 mg if required). Max 10 mg/24 h (5 mg/24 h if moderate-severe LF). Available intranasally[BNF/SPC].

ZOLPIDEM

'Non-benzodiazepine' hypnotic; see Zopiclone.

Use/CI/Caution/SE/Interactions: as Zopiclone but CI in psychotic illness, **P**.

Dose: 10 mg nocte. **NB: halve dose if LF (avoid if severe), severe RF or elderly.**

ZOMORPH Morphine sulphate capsules (10, 30, 60, 100 or 200 mg), equivalent in efficacy to Oramorph but SR: 12-hrly doses. See also Palliative Care section p. 189.

ZOPICLONE

Short-acting hypnotic (cyclopyrrolone): potentiates GABA pathways via same receptors as benzodiazepines (although isn't a benzodiazepine!): can also ⇒ dependence* and tolerance.

Use: insomnia (not long-term*).

CI: respiratory failure, sleep apnoea (severe), marked neuromuscular respiratory weakness (inc unstable MG), **L** (if severe**), **B**.

Caution: Ψ disorders, Hx of drug abuse*, muscle weakness, MG, **R/P/E**.

SE: *all rare*: GI upset, taste Δs, behavioural/Ψ disturbances (inc psychosis, aggression), hypersensitivity.

Interactions: Levels ↑by ritonavir, erythromycin and other enzyme inhibitors. Sedation ↑'d by other sedative medications and alcohol.

Dose: 7.5 mg nocte, ↑ing to 15 mg if necessary. **NB: halve dose if LF (avoid if severe**), severe RF or elderly.**

ZOTON see Lansoprazole; PPI.

ZYBAN see Bupropion; adjunct to smoking cessation.

Drug selection

ANTIBIOTICS

IMPORTANT POINTS

- The following *are only guides to a rational start to Rx*. Local organisms, sensitivities and prescribing preferences vary widely, and most UK hospitals now have antibiotic protocols: if unsure, consult your microbiology department/pharmacy.
- Empirical ('best guess') Rx is given unless stated otherwise.
- When deciding if 'severe' treatment is necessary, consider each individual's comorbidity and whether you have time to give simple Rx first and then add on or change if patient is not improving.
- Get as many appropriate cultures as possible *before* starting Rx; if unfamiliar with patient, check for recent culture results to aid choice of agent.
- If severe sepsis/shock (↓BP/urine output ± ↑lactate) see p. 251.

> ☠ It is essential to ask each patient *in person* about allergies before prescribing any antibiotics. Do not rely on notes or drug charts, which are often not complete or accurate. Remember: *if you prescribe it, you are liable!* If patient is unconscious, check notes thoroughly (or contact relatives/GP if time). Do not let an incident (or near-incident) be the way you learn this!☠.

PNEUMONIA

1. Community-acquired pneumonia

> *Severity assessment of community-acquired pneumonia in hospital*[1]
> Adapted with permission of BMJ Publishing Group from BTS guidelines. *Thorax* 2001; **56** (suppl IV) and 2004 update.
> *'CURB 65' score* – 1 point each for:
> - Confusion; MTS[2] ≤8/10 **or** *new* disorientation in time, place or person
> - Urea >7 mmol/l

- **Respiratory rate** ≥30/min
- **BP↓**: systolic <90 mmHg **or** diastolic ≤60 mmHg
- **65**: age ≥65 yrs

<2: Non-severe*; likely to be suitable for home treatment.
2: Severe** with *increased* risk of death; consider admission (or hospital supervised outpatient care) using clinical judgement.
>2: Severe** with *high* risk of death; admit and consider HDU/ITU (esp if ≥4).

[1]For assessment in the community use '*CRB 65*', which doesn't need blood test: 0 = likely to be suitable for home treatment; 1–2 = consider hospital referral; 3–4 = urgent hospital admission.
[2]MTS = (Abbreviated) Mental Test Score; see p. 269 for details.

Treatment:
*Non-severe***: amoxicillin 500 mg–1 g tds po ± clarithromycin*** 500 mg bd po (if admitted for clinical reasons).
*Severe****: co-amoxiclav 1.2 g tds iv + clarithromycin*** 500 mg bd iv ± flucloxacillin 1 g qds iv if *S. aureus* (Hx or epidemic of 'flu). ± rifampicin 600 mg bd po/iv if *Legionella* (do urinary Ag test).

- If no improvement, consider changing co-amoxiclav to tazocin (piperacillin + tazobactam).
- If risk factors, consider Rx for aspiration or TB as below.
- If penicillin hypersensitivity, use clarithromycin*** only.
- ***Clarithromycin is better tolerated than erythromycin (⇒ ↓GI upset); consult local protocol to check preference.

Causes of community-acquired pneumonia (UK adults)
Adapted with permission of BMJ Publishing Group from Lim WS, *et al. Thorax* 2001; **56**: 296–301.

- 48% *Streptococcus pneumoniae*: esp in winter or shelters/prison.
- 23% **viruses**: influenza (A ≫ B), RSV, rhinoviruses, adenoviruses.
- 15% *Chlamydia psittaci:* esp from animals, but only 20% from birds (less commonly *Chlamydia pneumoniae*, esp if long-term Hx and headache).
- 7% *Haemophilus influenzae.*

- 3%　***Mycoplasma pneumoniae:*** ↑s during 4-yrly epidemics.
- 3%　***Legionella pneumophila:*** ↑d if recent travel (esp Turkey, Spain).
- 2%　***Moraxella catarrhalis:*** ↑d in elderly.
- 1.5%　***Staphylococcus aureus:*** mostly post-influenza ∴ ↑s in winter.
- 1.4%　**Gram-negative infection:** *Escherichia coli, Pseudomonas, Klebsiella, Proteus, Serratia.*
- 1.1%　**Anaerobes:** e.g. *Bacteroides, Fusobacterium.*
- 0.7%　***Coxiella burnetii:*** ↑s in April–June and in sheep farmers.

NB: 25% are mixed aetiology (accounts for total of >100%).
In ≥20% of cases, causative pathogen is not identified.

The term 'atypical pathogens' is not considered useful by the BTS (refers to *Mycoplasma, Chlamydia, Coxiella, Legionella*) as there is no characteristic clinical presentation for the pneumonias they cause.

2. Hospital-acquired pneumonia
Non-severe: co-amoxiclav 625 mg tds po.
Severe: co-amoxiclav 1.2 g tds iv (or tazocin (piperacillin + tazobactam) 4.5 g tds iv if *Pseudomonas* suspected (or meropenem 1 g tds if penicillin allergy). DO NOT prescribe meropenem if history of anaphylactic or accelerated allergic reaction – discuss alternatives with microbiologist.
+ metronidazole 500 mg tds ivi if aspiration suspected. Now controversial.
+ gentamicin if septic shock or failure to improve.
MRSA: teicoplanin/vancomycin if confirmed colonisation/infection.

> *Causes of hospital-acquired pneumonia*
> Reproduced with permission from Hammersmith Hospitals NHS Trust Clinical Management Guidelines & Formulary 2001.
>
> - *Simple:* (w/in 7 days of admission): *H. influenzae, S. pneumoniae, S. aureus,* Gram-negative organisms (see top of page).
> - *Complicated*:* Gram-negative organisms (esp *P. aeruginosa*), *Acinetobacter,* MRSA.
> - *Anaerobic**:* *Bacteroides, Fusobacterium.*

- *Special situations:*
  1 Head trauma, coma, DM, RF: consider *S. aureus*.
  2 Mini-epidemics in hospitals: consider *Legionella*.

* > 7 days after admission, recent multiple antibiotics or complex medical Hx (e.g. recent ITU/
recurrent admissions or severe comorbidity).
**esp if risk of aspiration, recent abdominal surgery, bronchial obstruction/poor dentition.

3. Aspiration pneumonia
Treatment as for community- or hospital-acquired pneumonia, + metronidazole 500 mg tds ivi or 400 mg tds po.

4. Cavitating pneumonia
Co-amoxiclav 1.2 g tds iv (or flucloxacillin 1 g qds iv).
  NB: need to exclude TB with sputum/Heaf test ± pleural Bx, and consider septic emboli as a cause, e.g. from right-sided endocarditis. If MRSA suspected/confirmed use vancomycin iv plus rifampicin po.

'TANKS' Cause cavitation: **TB**, *Aspergillus*, *Nocardia*, *K*lebsiella, *S*. *aureus* (and *PS*eudomonas).

TB
Should normally be managed by respiratory or infectious disease physicians with expertise in this area.
  NB: Notify cases to public health authorities, and isolate potentially infectious inpatients.
  Rx normally comes in two phases:
- *Initial phase:* for 1st 2 months: ↓s bacterial load and covers all strains: Rifater* (**R**ifampicin + **I**soniazid + **P**yrazinamide) + **E**thambutol** = 'RIPE'.
- *Continuation phase:* for next 4 months (or longer if CNS involvement): Rifinah* (rifampicin + isoniazid) = 'RI'.
  If resistance to rifampicin/isoniazid known (or suspected), continue pyrazinamide = 'RIP'.
  - Consider pyridoxine 10 mg od po: ↓s isoniazid neuropathy[BNF].
  - Combined tablets* ⇒ ↑compliance and ease of prescribing.

– All doses are by weight; see BNF for details.
– All are hepatotoxic: check LFTs before and during Rx.
– **Ethambutol**** **is nephrotoxic and can** ⇒ **optic neuritis:** check U&Es and visual acuity before and during Rx. Alternative is streptomycin (also nephrotoxic), but both can be omitted if ↓risk of isoniazid resistance.
– **Corticosteroids** are usually added to this regimen from the start if meningeal or pericardial TB.

ACUTE BRONCHITIS

Rx not usually needed in previously healthy patients <60 yrs old.

- *Exacerbation of COPD:* 1st-line: doxycycline 200 mg od po. 2nd-line: amoxicillin (or co-amoxiclav).
- *Exacerbation of bronchiectasis:* co-amoxiclav 1.2 g tds iv (po if mild) or tazocin (piperacillin + tazobactam) 4.5 g tds iv (if severe, or if colonised with pseudomonas).
- *Cystic fibrosis:* ciprofloxacin 500 mg bd po (or 400 mg bd ivi) if *Pseudomonas* suspected. Otherwise try gentamicin + piperacillin until sensitivities known.

UPPER RESPIRATORY TRACT AND ENT INFECTIONS

- *Acute epiglottitis:* cefotaxime 1 g tds iv + metronidazole 500 mg tds ivi (or tazocin (piperacillin + tazobactam) 4.5 g tds iv). Ceftriaxone alone should suffice in children.
- *Pharyngitis/tonsillitis* (sore/'Strep' throat): penicillin V (phenoxy-methylpenicillin) 500 mg qds po if Hx of otitis media, confirmed group A Strep infection or 3 of the following 4 clues that infection is not viral: purulent tonsils, Hx of fever, lack of cough or cervical lymphadenopathy.
- *Sinusitis/otitis media:* amoxicillin 500 mg tds po if local pus or if does not resolve in 2–3 days (as would expect if viral aetiology).
- *Otitis externa:* mostly bacterial; give topical steroid plus antibiotic combination: Sofradex or Otomize. Less commonly fungal (look for black spores); give topical Otosporin or Neo-cortef. If does not resolve or evidence of perichondritis (inflamed pinna), cellulitis,

boils or local abscess, refer to ENT for specialist advice and consideration of systemic Rx (e.g. amoxicillin, co-amoxiclav, flucloxacillin) and local toilet (esp if fungal).

URINARY TRACT INFECTIONS

- *Simple UTI:* trimethoprim 200 mg bd po. Another option is nitrofurantoin 50–100 mg qds po (not suitable if RF).
- *Pyelonephritis (suspect if loin pain/systemic features):* cefotaxime 1 g tds iv. If no response within 24 h (and still no culture results), try co-amoxiclav 1.2 g tds iv + gentamicin.

Causes of UTIs
- Most caused by *E. coli* (70–80%).
- Remainder caused by Enterococci, or other Gram-negatives – e.g. *Proteus* (assoc. with stones), *Klebsiella, Serratia* or *Pseudomonas.*
- Staph saprophyticus seen in young women.
- Multi-resistant organisms more likely in catheterised or hospitalised patients.

GI INFECTIONS

Gastroenteritis
- Simple infections rarely need Rx; focus on rehydration and contact microbiology department if in doubt.
- *AAC (Clostridium difficile):* metronidazole 400 mg tds po and *stop other antibiotics if possible.* If no response after 4 days, change to vancomycin 125 mg qds po for 10–14 days.

Helicobacter pylori eradication: 'triple therapy'
Give 7-day course (for treatment failure consult BNF ± microbiology opinion).

1 *Antibiotic 1:* clarithromycin 500 mg bd po.
2 + *Antibiotic 2:* amoxicillin 1 g bd po (or metronidazole 400 mg bd; if used ↓clarithromycin dose to 250 mg bd).

3 + *Acid suppressant:* PPI; choose from omeprazole 20 mg bd, esomeprazole 20 mg bd, lansoprazole 30 mg bd, pantoprazole 40 mg bd or rabeprazole 20 mg bd.

MALARIA

Clues: fevers ($\pm$3-day cycles $\pm$ rigors), $\downarrow$Pt, $\downarrow$Hb, jaundice, $\uparrow$spleen/liver, travel (even >1 year previously).

  Always consult infectious diseases $\pm$ microbiology team if malaria suspected/confirmed.

If confirmed non-falciparum ('benign'):

- Chloroquine (as base; see below) dose 620 mg po, then 310 mg 6–8 h later, then 310 mg od 24 h later for 2 days (all doses of chloroquine as *base*). Follow, unless pregnant, with 14 days primaquine if *P. ovale* (15 mg od) or *P. vivax* (30 mg od) to kill parasites in the liver and prevent relapses (as a 'radical cure'). Primaquine dose: 30 mg od (*P. vivax*) or 15 mg od (*P. ovale*) for 14 days.

If falciparum ('malignant') or species mixed/unknown:
If seriously ill (e.g. $\downarrow$GCS), get senior help and give:

- Quinine (as salt; see below): load with 20 mg/kg ivi (max 1.4 g) over 4 h (NB: omit loading dose if quinine, quinidine or mefloquine given in past 12 h.) Then, 8 h after the start of the loading dose, give 10 mg/kg (max 700 mg) ivi over 4 h every 8 h for up to 7 days ($\downarrow$doses to 5–7 mg/kg if RF or >48 h if iv Rx needed), changing to oral quinine (600 mg tds of salt) once able to swallow and retain tablets to complete a 7-day course.
- Doxycycline 200 mg od po (clindamycin 450 mg tds po if pregnant) with or following quinine course for 7 days.
- Consider artesunate or artemether if patient has been to quinine-resistant areas of SE Asia: get specialist advice.

If stable, normal GCS, and able to swallow and retain tablets:

- Quinine: 600 mg tds po for 7 days followed by doxycycline or clindamycin. Proguanil + atovaquone (Malarone), artemether + lumefantrine (Riamet) are alternatives (Rx for 3 days only) to quinine which only need to be taken for 3 days and don't need any subsequent drugs.

> 🐍 Quinine doses here are as 'salt' (quinine hydrochloride, dihydrochloride or sulphate). Choloroquine doses are as 'base' (i.e. the chloroquine component of the total drug compound). Specify salt or base on the prescription: don't confuse salt or base doses as they are not equivalent.

MENINGITIS

Empirical Rx (until results of LP known – esp Gram stain).

- Cefotaxime 2 g qds ivi: Rx of choice for *N. meningitides* (aka meningococcus; commonest cause in UK adults). If Hx of severe hypersensitivity (e.g. anaphylaxis) to cephalosporins (or penicillins as 10% also hypersensitive to cephalosporins) consider chloramphenicol 1 g tds/qds iv (can ↑ to 100 mg/kg/day$^{SPC/BNF}$); if allergy (but not anaphylaxis) use meropenem 2 g tds iv.

Consider:

- Ampicillin 2 g 4-hrly ivi + gentamicin iv if *Listeria* suspected, e.g. immunosuppression or indicative CSF: Gram-positive bacilli.
- Aciclovir 10 mg/kg over 1 h tds ivi if HSV encephalitis suspected, e.g. more prominent confusion, behavioural Δs and seizures.
- TB Rx as for pneumonia, and discuss with Infectious Diseases/ Microbiology: if risk factors or suggestive CSF findings (↑LØ, ↑protein, ↓glucose). Negative CSF stains for acid-fast bacilli do NOT exclude the diagnosis; if clinical suspicion high Rx shouldn't be delayed while awaiting microbiological confirmation.

Causes of meningitis in the UK
Common:
- *N. meningitidis*, serotype B: majority (70–80%) of cases.
- *N. meningitidis*, serotype C: ↓ing secondary to vaccine.

- *N. meningitidis*, serotype A: ↓ing again (had been ↓ing).
- *S. pneumoniae*: stable incidence.

Rarer:
- Gram-negative bacilli (esp in neonates).
- *Listeria monocytogenes*: esp neonates, age >60yr, ↓immunity.
- *H. influenzae*, type b: ↓ing secondary to vaccine.

Don't forget:
- Viral: HSV/HZV, EBV, HIV, mumps: esp if encephalitic (↓GCS). Less commonly entero/echo/Coxsackie/polio viruses.
- TB, other bacteria, e.g. *Borrelia*: esp if ↓immunity/HIV.
- Fungi: *Cryptococcus, Candida*: esp if ↓immunity/HIV.
- Group B *Streptococcus*: predominantly in neonates.
- *S. aureus*: if neurosurgery, trauma or ventricular shunt.

EYE INFECTIONS

- *Conjunctivitis* (only Rx if prolonged/atypical): chloramphenicol 0.5% 1 drop qds.
- *Orbital cellulitis*:
  - If preseptal (lids only) ⇒ oral co-amoxiclav, can be managed as outpatient with close observation.
  - If retro-orbital admit for iv Rx (e.g. ceftriaxone + metronidazole).
- *Corneal ulcer*: Needs urgent ophthalmology referral. Ofloxacin 0.3% 1 drop hrly day and night for 48 hrs then hrly daytime; specialist advice required for length or Rx.
  - Only give once scrape taken for Gram stain/culture.
  - Suspect in contact lens wearer with painful red eye ⇒ refer to ophthalmologist urgently.
  - Don't allow patients to self administer topical anaesthetic for analgesia as ⇒ epithelium to slough ☠.
- *Blepharitis:* Lid margin/eyelash scrubs only. If severe or lid hygiene alone insufficient ⇒ Maxitrol ointment (dexamethasone 0.1% & neomycin 0.35%) applied to lashes BD for 1 month in addition to

lid hygiene. Artificial tears (hypromellose) can also be used to reduce symptoms.
- *Acute chalazion/Stye:* can be managed with regular warm compresses to burst cyst (antibiotics not required). If concern that early cellulitis ⇒ oral antibiotics may also be given (see above).

CELLULITIS

- Mild (e.g. Venflon site infection): co-amoxiclav 625 mg tds po or flucloxacillin 500 mg qds po.
- Severe: benzylpenicillin 1.2 g iv 4–6-hrly + flucloxacillin 1 g qds iv.
  - + metronidazole 500 mg tds ivi if suspect anaerobes, e.g. abdominal wound.
  - + consider vancomycin 1 g bd ivi if confirmed MRSA colonisation/ infection.

BONE AND JOINT INFECTIONS

Osteomyelitis: suspect in any postoperative joint or deep DM ulcer.

- Flucloxacillin 1–2 g qds iv + fusidic acid 500 mg tds po (can give iv in severe cases, but is poorly tolerated and often not required; see main drugs section for doses). *Staph aureus* is usual cause, but in spinal infection consider also Gram-negatives, and discuss with Microbiology.
- If MRSA suspected consult local guidelines ± microbiologist.
- In osteomyelitis associated with chronic ulcers, co-amoxiclav 1.2 g tds iv should be given instead of flucloxacillin.
- If penicillin allergy give clindamycin 600 mg qds iv.

Septic arthritis: suspect if sudden-onset pain/inflammation.

- Treatment as osteomyelitis, but consider changing after urgent Gram stain, e.g. to iv 3rd-generation cephalosporin (e.g. cefotaxime, ceftriaxone) if *H. influenzae* suspected (Gram-negative bacilli, esp in children). Suspect *Salmonella* in sickle cell disease or TB/ fungi if immunocompromised.

PUO

No routine antibiotics indicated, but suspect and exclude abdominal abscess, TB, Ca (esp abdominal/haematological) and other causes.

> **Causes of PUO**
> - Abdominal abscess: liver, subphrenic, pelvic.
> - Other infection: UTI, TB, malaria, infective endocarditis, bone infection, virus (EBV, CMV, HIV).
> - Autoimmune: rheumatoid arthritis, Still's disease, PMR, sarcoid, PAN, SLE/connective tissue disease.
> - Cancer: lymphoma, leukaemia, solid tumours (esp abdominal).
> - Drugs: almost any (inc drugs of abuse), often assoc w ↑EØ.
> - Other: PEs, haematomas, alcoholic hepatitis, FMF.
>
> NB: up to 25% of cases remain unexplained.

FEBRILE NEUTROPENIA

If temperature 38°C for ≥2 h (or ≥38.5°C for ≥1 h) and no clues as to the fever's aetiology, give:

- *For 1st/2nd episodes:* gentamicin 5 mg/kg od iv + Tazocin 4.5 g tds iv (use ceftazidime 2 g tds iv if penicillin allergy).
- *For persistent or recurrent fever at any later stage:* call haematologist/oncologist ± microbiologist on call for advice.

> NB: Always do full septic screen before giving/prescribing antibiotics: blood, urine and any other appropriate cultures (e.g. sputum, stool, central/other lines) ± CXR.

HYPERTENSION MANAGEMENT

Adapted with permission of NICE www.nice.org.uk/guidance/CG127 (2011 revision).

When to treat: depends on severity and other factors:

Severity	Clinic BP[1]		ABPM[2] or HBPM[3]	Drug therapy[4]
Normotensive	<140/90	*OR*	<135/85	No
Stage 1	≥140/90	*AND*	≥135/85	Consider[5]
Stage 2	≥160/100	*AND*	≥150/95	Yes
Severe	SBP ≥180 OR DBP ≥110			Yes, immediate

1. All measurements are in mmHg. If 1st clinic BP ≥140/90, repeat. If 2nd measurement much lower that 1st take 3rd reading; lowest of 2nd & 3rd is taken as clinic BP. Clinic BP persistly ≥140/90 should be confirmed by ABPM/HBPM unless ≥180 OR 110. 2. Ambulatory BP monitoring; average of ≥14 daytime readings. 3. Home BP monitoring; average of ≥4 days a.m. & evening readings, excluding 1st days readings. 4. Encourage lifestyle modifications *for all* ↑BP: ↓salt, ↓Wt, ↓alcohol, stop smoking, ↑exercise, ↑fresh fruit/vegetables, ↓intake of total and unsaturated fat. For Stage 1 without CVD or target organ damage*, these measures can be tried before drug therapy. 5. Indicated in those <80 years old if established CVD or DM, or evidence of target organ damage*, or 10-yr CVD risk ≥20% (see risk charts at back of BNF or at http://www.bhsoc.org/Cardiovascular_Risk_Charts_and_Calculators.stm).
*HF, established IHD, CVA/TIA, chronic kidney disease (CKD, ↓GFR, ↑creatinine or proteinuria/microalbuminuria), hypertensive/diabetic retinopathy or LVH.

🕱 See p. 244 for Dx and Mx of accelerated HTN🕱 .

Aim for: Clinic BP ≤140/90 mmHg if <80 y.o.; <150/90 if ≥80 y.o. If CKD ≤140/90mmHg. If DM or CKD and >1g/24h proteinuria (urinary albumin:creatinine ratio >70 mg/mmol or protein:creatinine ratio >100 mg/mmol) ≤ 130/80 mmHg. Consider ABPM/HBPM in those with white coat effect. If target not achieved with Step 1, progress to Step 2 etc.

Primary causes: look for and exclude (esp if treatable), e.g. RAS, Conn's (1° hyperaldosteronism), ↑Ca^{2+}, Cushing's, phaeo (esp if variable BP, headaches, sweats, palpitations), oestrogen-containing contraceptive pills and recreational drugs (e.g. alcohol, cocaine, amphetamines).

NB: stress (inc 'white-coat HTN'), recreational drug use and withdrawal (esp alcohol) are common temporary causes.

Important points:

- Make a *written* Rx plan for (other) doctors, nurses and patient. Include target BP and how Rx should change if it is not achieved.
- Age/ethnic origin influence response to drugs (see table below).
- A single agent is rarely successful at achieving target BP. Rather than ↑ing doses, add 2nd and 3rd agents, which often work in an additive or complementary fashion, esp if table below used.
- Exclude/minimise dietary salt and NSAID (inc unrecognized 'over-the-counter') use, as reason for poor treatment response.

Choice of drug: rational combination therapy[NICE/2011]

Step	Younger(<55 yrs) and non-black		Older (≥55 yrs) or black[1]
1	A[2]		C[3]
2		A[2] + C[3]	
3		A[2] + C + D	
4		Resistant hypertension[4]	

1. Black = African (not Asian) origin. 2. β-Blockers are an alternative to ACE-i/ARBS but see notes below. 3. If C not suitable (e.g. presence or risk of LVF, intolerance, oedema) offer D [thiazide-like diuretic]. 4. Ensure on optimal/best tolerated doses of A + C + D. Check adherence to lifestyle advice. If K+ ≤4.5 mmol/L add spironolactone (e.g. 25 mg od). ☠ CKD, due to risk of ↑K+. If K+ >4.5 mmol/L consider higher dose thiazide diuretic (e.g. chlorthalidone 50–200 mg od), α-blocker or β-blocker. Consider missed 1° cause ±specialist referral.

☺ good for, ☹ avoid/caution, ☠ *beware!*

- *A = ACE-i*, e.g. ramipril initially 2.5 mg od (1.25 mg if elderly or CKD). ☺ CKD (but *with caution!*), HF, DM, IHD. ☹PVD (as assoc with RAS*)☠. Pregnancy, bilateral RAS*. (*Must monitor U&Es 2 wks after starting, then regularly, esp if vasculopathy or CKD*). **Angiotensin** II receptor blockers (ARBs) are preferred to ACE-I in Blacks. Also use if ACE-i not tolerated (esp dt dry cough). Use low cost ARBs. Monitor as for ACE-i. Do not combine ACE-i + ARB.

- *B = β-blocker*, e.g. atenolol 50 mg od. ☺ younger patients with ↑sympathetic drive or childbearing potential, IHD (post-MI/angina), chronic stable LVF, intolerance to ACE-i or ARB. If used for Step 1, add C for Step 2 (in preference to D) to ↓risk of DM. ☹ dyslipidaemia, PVD, DM (unless also IHD), if on diltiazem. ☠ asthma/COPD, HB, acute LVF, if on verapamil.

- *C = Ca²⁺-channel blocker:* dihydropyridines such as amlodipine 5 mg or nifedipine LA (e.g. Adalat LA 20–30 mg od) usually 1st-line. ☹ oedema, polyuria. ☠ aortic stenosis, recent ACS.

- If IHD 'rate-limiting' types (verapamil, diltiazem) often preferred. ☠ HF, HB, if on other rate-limiting drugs (esp β-blockers).

- *D = thiazide-like diuretic*, e.g. indapamide SR 1.5 mg od or chlorthalidone 25mg od. ☺ oedema/HF. ☹ dyslipidaemia. ☠ gout. If patient on conventional thiazide diuretic (e.g. bendroflumethiazide) and BP controlled, continue this.

NB: only starting doses are given; see main drugs section or SPCs/BNF for doses thereafter.

ASTHMA

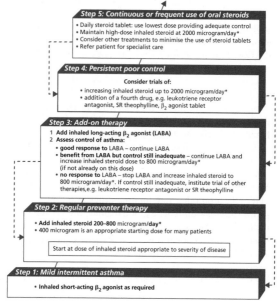

Step 5: Continuous or frequent use of oral steroids
- Daily steroid tablet: use lowest dose providing adequate control
- Maintain high-dose inhaled steroid at 2000 microgram/day*
- Consider other treatments to minimise the use of steroid tablets
- Refer patient for specialist care

Step 4: Persistent poor control

Consider trials of:
- increasing inhaled steroid up to 2000 microgram/day*
- addition of a fourth drug, e.g. leukotriene receptor antagonist, SR theophylline, β_2 agonist tablet

Step 3: Add-on therapy
1 Add inhaled long-acting β_2 agonist (LABA)
2 Assess control of asthma:
- good response to LABA – continue LABA
- benefit from LABA but control still inadequate – continue LABA and increase inhaled steroid dose to 800 microgram/day* (if not already on this dose)
- no response to LABA – stop LABA and increase inhaled steroid to 800 microgram/day*. If control still inadequate, institute trial of other therapies,e.g. leukotriene receptor antagonist or SR theophylline

Step 2: Regular preventer therapy
- Add inhaled steroid 200–800 microgram/day*
- 400 microgram is an appropriate starting dose for many patients

Start at dose of inhaled steroid appropriate to severity of disease

Step 1: Mild intermittent asthma
- Inhaled short-acting β_2 agonist as required

*Beclometasone or budesonide (NB: fluticasone equivalent doses are half this).

Figure 1 BTS guidelines for management of asthma in adults. Adapted with permission of BMJ group from *Thorax* 2008; **63** (suppl 4): iv1–iv121 (revised 2011).

Patients should start treatment at the step most appropriate to the initial severity of their asthma. Check concordance and technique at every step and reconsider diagnosis if response to treatment is unexpectedly poor. Remember to move down (as well as up) the ladder to find and maintain lowest controlling step.

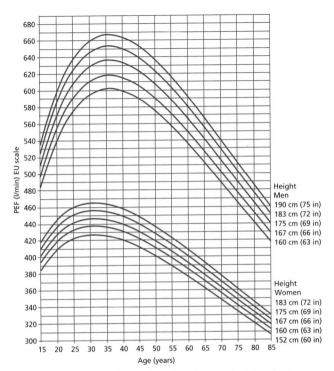

Figure 2 Peak expiratory flow (PEF) predictor for normal adults using European standard 'EU' (EN 13826) scale. Adapted with permission of BMJ group from Gregg I, Nunn AJ. *BMJ* 1989; **298**: 1098, corrected to the EN 13826: 2003 scale values by Clement Clarke International Ltd.

ANALGESIA

Choice of analgesic:

General rules
- Look for/treat reversible causes and reassess cause at each step.
- Regular Rx ↓s relapses *but always review to check whether still needed.*
- If pain ↓s, 'step down' and ensure adequate prn analgesia in case ↑s again.
- Pain has many adverse medical fx and is rarely refractory to the correct Rx.
- If pain persists, get senior or specialist help (e.g. anaesthetist or pain team).

- All opioids can ⇒ constipation, respiratory depression and ↓GCS (esp if elderly or RF – even low doses). Can also ⇒ coma if LF.
- All NSAIDs can ⇒ PU (related to strength of drug and length of Rx. Consider PPI or changing to COX2 inhibitor^NICE) Can also ⇒ AKI if fluid depleted (∴rehydrate 1st or avoid).

Step 4
- Strong opioid:
  iv if acute (e.g. morphine)
  po if chronic (e.g. *oramorph*)
  sc in palliative care: see p. 184

Step 3
- High dose weak opioid e.g.:
  – dihydrocodeine 30 mg qds
  – tramadol 50–100 mg qds (also has 5HT fx: ↓SEs for same analgesia)

Step 2
- Compound prep. of paracetamol with low dose weak opioid (e.g. cocodamol or codydramol) or weak opioid alone (e.g. dihydrocodeine)

Step 1
- **Simple analgesia:** paracetamol 1 g qds usually 1st-line as few SEs.

  NSAIDs 2nd-line; 1st line if predominant inflammatory component, e.g.:
  – Ibuprofen 200–400 mg tds po for mild pain.
  – Diclofenac (*Voltarol*) 50 mg tds im/po or 75 mg SR bd im/po or 100 mg pr (max 150 mg/day) for moderate pain (esp good postoperatively).

- **Consider specialist analgesia** according to cause, e.g. buscopan for colic, colchicine for gout, antacids for reflux, GTN for angina. For neuropathic pain try amitriptyline, gabapentin or pregabalin.

Figure 3 Analgesia ladder. Based on WHO pain relief ladder for cancer pain.

Important points for postoperative patients:
- Oral route often ineffective *for all operations* (due to gastric stasis).
- Epidural anaesthesia (EDA) and patient-controlled analgesia (PCA) normally provide maximal opiates (as well as other drugs)

∴ beware of giving more. Consider NSAID and get advice from anaesthetist if this does not work.

- Consider local/regional anaesthesia.

PALLIATIVE CARE AND SUBCUTANEOUS PUMPS

- Underprescribed due to stigma of being a 'final measure': ensure good communication with patient, relatives and nurses as to reasons for use.
- Gives smooth symptom control, esp for pain, but also useful for other symptoms, e.g. nausea, xs secretions, agitation. Good if unable to take po medications, avoids cannulation, only single 24 h prescription needed (no delays in drug administration on busy wards).
- Palliative care, Macmillan and hospital pain teams will help if unsure of the indications or how to set up these pumps.

CONTENTS OF SUBCUTANEOUS PUMP

4 *Diamorphine (or morphine sulphate)*: calculate dose needed for 24 h prescription from the past 24 hours' requirements (if variable, look at longer-term trend). If taking other opioids, use the following *rough* guide:

1 mg diamorphine sc/im = 1.5 mg morphine sc/im
= 3 mg morphine po
= 15 mg tramadol po
= 35 mg codeine po/im

(For conversion from fentanyl, see its entry in main drugs section.)

NB: these equivalent doses only apply for the specific route(s) of each drug stated, as bioavailability can vary widely with routes. Also, it does not take into account duration of action, although this can be ignored if 24 h requirements for each drug are calculated. At high opioid doses, conversion factors become less reliable – err on the conservative side and gradually titrate up.

5 Antiemetic: choose from (generally start at lowest dose):
- Metoclopramide 30–90 mg/24 h: (esp for promotility fx slow gastric emptying; but CI if GI obstruction with abdominal pain!).
- Haloperidol 0.5–5 mg/24 h: good general antiemetic.
- Cyclizine 50 mg tds sc/po/24 h: good if cause unknown or multifactorial.
- Levomepromazine 6.25–12.5 mg/24 h. Good if cause unknown or multifactorial (↑doses to 25–50 mg/h if sedation needed and patient not ambulant.)

6 Optional extras:
- Drugs to ↓respiratory secretions:
  – glycopyrronium 0.6–1.2 mg/24 h.
  – hyoscine hydrobromide 0.6–2.4 mg/24 h: normally sedative but can ⇒ paradoxical agitation. ↑risk of seizures.
- Sedatives, e.g. midazolam 10–80 mg/24 h if restlessness or agitation is the solitary symptom. Consider levomepromazine if not responsive to midazolam. Care/↓dose if elderly, respiratory depression, benzodiazepine-naive.

> *Compatibility of drugs in syringe drivers*
> It is advised that only two or three drugs are used per syringe driver. All antiemetics listed above are compatible with diamorphine and morphine. For addition of 'optional extras', see table below; for all other combinations, check with the hospital pharmacy or drug information office. Out-of-hours authoritative information on compatibility (and other palliative care prescribing issues) can be found at the excellent website www.palliativedrugs.com.

Compatibility* of specific three-drug combinations: diamorphine and antiemetic and one other 'optional extra'drug.

Diamorphine *plus*	Glycopyrronium	Hyoscine *hydrobromide*	Midazolam
Metoclopramide	Not recommended	Not recommended	Compatible*
Haloperidol	Compatible*	Compatible*	Compatible*
Levomepromazine	Compatible*	Compatible*	Compatible*

*Compatibility is restricted to usual dose ranges of the drugs.

EXAMPLE PRESCRIPTION

Prescribe each drug individually in the 'regular prescriptions' section of the drug chart, as shown here:

DATE/ TIME	INFUSION FLUID	VOL-UME	ADDITIVES IF ANY DRUG AND DOSE	RATE OF ADMIN	DURA-TION	DR'S SIGNATURE	TIME START-ED	TIME COMP-LETED	SET UP BY SIG-NATURE	BATCH No.
08/01	Water for injection	+	DIAMORPHINE 60 mg			TH				
		+	METOCLOPRAMIDE 30 mg							
Make up to syringe length of 48 mm to run subcutaneously via syringe driver at 2 mm per hour over 24 h										

Figure 4 Example drug chart of diamorphine subcutaneous pump. *NB: 60 mg diamorphine/24 h is* **example dose**; individual patient needs will vary (see above).

> *Graseby syringe drivers: mm (instead of ml) per unit time*
> This type of syringe driver is common in the UK (esp in specialist palliative care settings). Infusions are given in millimetres (mm) rather than millilitres (ml) per unit time. There are 2 types: for each unit on the 'rate' dial, the MS16 (blue) delivers 2 mm/h, but the MS26 (green) delivers 48 mm/day.
> Examples of prescriptions of a syringe to be given over 24 h:
>
> - **MS16:** 'Diamorphine 60 mg over 24 h as subcutaneous infusion via syringe driver. Mix with water for injection to a length of 48 mm in syringe, set at rate of 2 mm/h.'
> - **MS26:** 'Diamorphine 60 mg over 24 h as subcutaneous infusion via syringe driver. Mix with water for injection to a length of 48 mm in syringe, set at rate of 48 mm/24 h.'
>
> ☠ Confusing mm with ml or confusing the 2 types of driver can lead to significant differences in rate of drug delivery ☠.

GENERAL POINTERS IN CHRONIC PAIN/ PALLIATIVE CARE

- *Laxatives:* give with opiates as Px rather than later as Rx.
- *Simple analgesia:* do not forget as often effective, e.g. regular paracetamol.

- *Breakthrough analgesia:* always write up in case regular medications become insufficient. Oral opiates (e.g. Oramorph) often best; 1/6 of regular 24-h opiate equivalent dose is usually sufficient. If ↓GCS or ↓swallow add sc or iv drugs (e.g. morphine).
- *Fentanyl patches:* smooth pain control w/o multiple injections or tablets (just change patch every 3rd day). Also less constipating. ☠ Only use if stable opioid requirements; long action means dose overestimation can be fatal. ☠
- *Steroids:* consider for nausea, as pain adjuvant (esp liver capsule pain), and for short-term Rx of ↓appetite: get specialist help.
- *Always consider new causes of pain/distress,* esp if patient unable to give Hx: often treatable, iatrogenic or can be disguised/made worse by more analgesia, e.g. opiate-induced constipation, patient positioning, UTI, urinary retention, mental anguish (esp 'unfinished business'), pathological fractures.

Commonly missed problems

- ↑Ca^{2+}: esp consider if confusion and constipation (other symptoms: 'bones, stones, groans and psychic moans'); see p. 259 for Mx.
- *Spinal cord compression:* ↑back pain, sensory/sphincter disturbance, limb weakness – *can be treated* with immediate high-dose steroids (e.g. dexamethasone phosphate 12–16 mg iv stat then 8 mg po bd) and radiotherapy; refer urgently to oncologist.

ANTIEMETICS

Commonly used 1st-line/narrow-spectrum antiemetics (see also Palliative Care section, p. 189).

General rules

- Look for/treat reversible causes (see below).
- Reassess causes at each step.
- Start sc/im/iv switching to po when able.
- Consider sc pump if chronic uncontrolled (see p. 180).
- Don't stop Rx unless cause removed.

Step 4
- Combine different antiemetics: aim to progressively block different receptors.

Step 3
- Try levomepromazine or a $5HT_3$ antagonist (e.g. ondansetron).

Step 2
- Try alternative or add 2nd narrow-spectrum agent.
- Consider dexamethasone if cause is brain tumour (or other cause of ICP) or chemotherapy.

Step 1
- Start narrow-spectrum (1st line) drug: choose most appropriate agent from the table on next page.

Figure 5 Antiemetic ladder – designed for cancer patients; steps 3 and 4 are rarely needed in other settings.

Causes of nausea
- *Drugs:* esp opiates, chemotherapy/cytotoxics, antibiotics (esp erythromycin, metronidazole). Commonly also dopamine agonists, antidepressants (esp fluoxetine), theophyllines, colchicine, $FeSO_4$ and acutely amiodarone/digoxin.
- *GI:* constipation, but also surgical (obstruction, peritonism) and medical (oesophagitis, gastritis, PU) causes.
- *Neurological:* migraine, ↑ICP (esp tumour), meningitis, Menière's, labyrinthitis.
- *Metabolism:* ↑Ca^{2+} (also ↓Na^+, ↑K^+), DKA, AKI, Addison's.
- *Infection:* gastroenteritis, UTI (often presenting symptom), respiratory infections.
- *Other:* post-operative, pregnancy, MI (esp inferior, often ↓pain if DM/elderly).

Class	Example	Good for	Beware
Phenothiazine (D_2 antagonist)	**Haloperidol** 0.5–1.5 mg sc/po	Opiates, general anaesthetic, postoperative, chemo-/radio-therapy (if mild), 1st choice in LF	⇒ ↑ prolactin, extrapyramidal fx, ↓s seizure threshold, ↓BP
Butyrophenone (D_2 antagonist)	**Levomepromazine** 6.25–25 mg od or bd po/sc/iv	Broad spectrum: useful when cause unclear/multifactorial	⇒ sedation, ↓BP ↓s seizure threshold
Benzamine (D_2 antagonist)	**Metoclopramide** 10(–20) mg tds po/sc/im/iv (Maxolon)	(GI causes ↑s GI motility*), migraine, drugs (esp opiates)	⇒ ↑ prolactin, extrapyramidal fx, ⊗ CI if GI obstruction ⊗ *
Benzamine (D_2 antagonist)	**Domperidone** 10–20 mg tds po or 30–60 mg bd pr (*not iv or im*)	Parkinson's disease**, morning-after pill, chemotherapy	⇒ ↑ prolactin, but minimal sedation and extrapyramidal fx**
Antihistamines	**Cyclizine** 50 mg tds po/sc/im/iv	GI obstruction*/postoperative N&V, vestibular/labyrinthine disorders. Antiemetic of choice in LF	⇒ Antimuscarinic fx (esp sedation). Avoid in IHD(↓s beneficial cardiodynamic fx of opiates)
5HT$_3$ antagonists	**Ondansetron** 4–8 mg bd po/ im/iv (16 mg od pr) **Granisetron Tropisetron**	Severe/resistant cases (esp chemo-/radio-therapy)	Minimal side effects:headache, constipation, dizziness

*Prokinetic fx of metoclopramide by anticholinergic drugs (see p. 233), esp cyclizine if also used in this setting.

**Extrapyramidal fx possible with all D2 antagonists (see p. 236) but less so with domperidone.

ALCOHOL WITHDRAWAL

A 'detox' programme comprises the following components:

1. PREVENTION OF AGITATION, SEIZURES AND DELIRIUM TREMENS

Give a long-acting benzodiazepine in a tapered regimen as follows:

Alcohol withdrawal regimen. Courtesy of Professor
H. Ghodse, St George's Hospital.

Day	Chlordiazepoxide	OR	Diazepam
1	30 mg qds		15 mg qds
2	30 mg tds		10 mg qds
3	20 mg tds		10 mg tds
4	20 mg bd		5 mg qds
5	10 mg bd		5 mg tds
6	10 mg od		5 mg bd
7	10 mg prn		5 mg od

These are only suggested initial average regimens
Requirements vary considerably with severity of symptoms and
previous experience of or tolerance to benzodiazepines. Regular dose
review and prescription of prn doses is essential. Some patients may
require a longer stabilisation period before starting to reduce doses.
Ideal regimens involve an initial 24-h assessment of prn doses, but
require adequate training and time of staff to monitor closely and
ensure no under- (or over-) treatment occurs. Start with dose of 20–40
mg chlordiazepoxide or 10–20 mg diazepam and add up doses used in
1st 24 h, then reduce by 1/5th (–1/7th) per day for 5(–7) days.

- Chlordiazepoxide usually 1st line, but diazepam preferred if Hx
  of seizures (esp if occurred in context of alcohol withdrawal).
- If significant liver failure (e.g. ↑AST or ALT), consider
  shorter-acting benzodiazepines such as oxazepam or lorazepam at
  equivalent doses (see p. 230); avoids xs metabolite build up and
  sedation (but marginal ↑seizure risk).

- Only start once acute alcohol intoxication has resolved as benzodiazepines are contraindicated in this state.

2. THIAMINE (VIT B1) AND OTHER SUPPLEMENTS

For Px or Rx of suspected Wernicke's encephalopathy (WE): must give before patient receives carbohydrate load po or iv, which can precipitate WE.

☠ ∴ Take particular care if hypoglycaemic and iv glucose needed! ☠

- **Parenteral (iv or im) thiamine:** e.g. Pabrinex (contains other B and C vits); prescribe as '1 pair Pabrinex vials' or 'Pabrinex 1 and 2'. British Association of Psychopharmacology guidelines 2004 recommend:
  - If WE established (or *suspected*; see note box below): 2 pairs tds iv (or im) for 3 days, then 1 pair od for 3–5 days.
  - If high risk of WE (malnourished/chronic severe abuse):1 pair od iv im for 3–5 days.
  - If low risk of WE no parenteral treatment needed.

☠ Pabrinex *can* ⇒ *anaphylaxis*
∴ ensure resus facilities at hand. NB: ↑risk if given iv too quickly; ensure mixture of both vials either given as injection over ≥ 10 min or as infusion (with 50–100 ml saline) over ≥ 30 min ☠ .

- Oral vitamins and supplements.
  - Thiamine 100 mg bd/tds po; should be given for 1 month if no parenteral treatment required.
  - Multivitamins 1 tablet/day long-term; cheap and potentially important if future diet unlikely to be good.

> *Wernicke's encephalopathy*
> Caused by thiamine deficiency and often missed; only 10% have classical triad of confusion, ataxia and eye signs (ophthalmoplegia or nystagmus; seen in only 30% of cases). Suspect diagnosis if any evidence of chronic alcohol misuse and any one of: acute confusion, ataxia, ophthalmoplegia, ↓BP + ↓temp, ↓GCS or ↓memory. If unsure whether intoxication or WE causing any of that, always assume it is WE and give treatment. Rarely WE is caused by other malnutrition, e.g. malabsorption, eating disorders, protracted vomiting, CRF, AIDS and other drug misuse. NB: ↓Mg^{2+} can ⇒ Rx refractory WE ∴ check ± correct Mg^{2+}.

3. MAINTENANCE OF ABSTINENCE

It is essential to:

- Encourage abstinence and refer to local alcohol liaison nurse (if available) ± addiction services.
- Treat depression and try to arrange adequate social support.

Consider the following as aids:

- *Acamprosate:* modulates alcohol withdrawal fx & limits −ve reinforcement of drinking cessation ⇒ ↓cravings and ↓relapse rate.
- *Disulfiram:* ⇒ unpleasant symptoms if alcohol consumed.
- *Naltrexone:* ↓s pleasurable fx of alcohol and ↓s craving and relapse rate. Specialist use only (not yet licensed in UK for this indication).

ANTIDEPRESSANTS

Depression is common, esp in chronic illness/inpatients (50%). It is easy to miss, responds to treatment and has impact on medical outcomes. Be vigilant for its presence ± screen (e.g. PHQ-9 screening tool). NICE recommends asking if during the last month the patient has been bothered by 'Feeling down, depressed or hopeless?' *or* 'Having little interest or pleasure in doing things?'.

If suspected, establish ICD-10 diagnosis by enquiring for the following 10 symptoms:

1. Depressed mood
2. Energy loss: $\Rightarrow$ fatiguability and $\downarrow$activity
3. Pleasure, interest and enjoyment loss (=anhedonia)
4. Retardation (psychomotor). NB: atypically $\Rightarrow$ agitation
5. Eating Δ: $\downarrow$appetite/wt. NB: atypically can $\uparrow$
6. Sleep disturbance (early morning waking)
7. Suicidal/self-harm thoughts
8. I'm a failure; loss of confidence/self-esteem
9. Only me to blame (guilt/unworthiness)
10. No concentration or attention

1st 3 are 'core'* symptoms: ≥ 2 required for diagnosis.

NICE recommendations

Severity	ICD-10 Symptoms(≥ 2 core*)	Action
Mild	4	Watchful waiting + consider self help/psychological Rx
Moderate	5–6	Consider antidepressant and/or CBT
Severe	$\geq 7(\pm$ psychotic symptoms)	Antidepressant $\pm$ CBT

- If moderate/severe depression treat for 6 months beyond recovery and review need for further treatment.
- Treat for ≥ 2 years if ≥ 2 depressive episodes with significant functional impairment in the recent past.
- Pharmacological treatment should be combined with other psychological interventions where possible, e.g. cognitive behaviour interventions.

> ☠ Beware prescribing in the depressive phase of bipolar disorder (screen for previous mania/hypomania); risk of inducing mania (esp with venlafaxine and paroxetine) ☠

Give information sheet on antidepressants (e.g. http://www.rcpsych.ac.uk/mentalhealthinformation/mentalhealthproblems/depression/antidepressants.aspx) highlighting risk of discontinuation syndrome if stopped abruptly (see p. 235).

TREATMENT RESISTANCE/POOR TOLERANCE

1 Check compliance/adequate dose.
2 ↑ to max dose unless limited by side effects.
3 Change class if adequate trial given for ≥6 weeks.
4 Consider specialist input: trial of MAOI, combination of antidepressants or augmentation with lithium or atypical antipsychotic.

☠ Monitor for increased suicidal ideation or development of hypomania/mania ☠

Class	Drug	☺ Good for/reasons to prescribe	☹ Bad for/reasons to avoid		
SSRI	Fluoxetine	Risks for OD[5] (safer); Anxiety; OCD; Few SEs	Risk of abrupt stopping (long t₁/₂); Children[8]	Sexual SEs (↓libido, impotence etc); agitation (or akathisia); risk of osteoporosis with long-term use	Polypharmacy (↑interactions)
	Paroxetine				Inconsistent use[11] or <25 years old[12]
	(Es)[1] Citalopram				
	Sertraline		Polypharmacy[9] or IHD		
SARI	Trazodone	Insomnia		(Postural)hypotension	
NaSSA	Mirtazapine	Insomnia,[6] sexual dysfunction[4] or polypharmacy[9]		Concern about weight gain	
TCA	Amitriptyline	Insomnia (esp initial, i.e. getting off to sleep); chronic pain (neuralgia, migraine, back pain etc)		Risks for OD[5] (less safe); (Postural) hypotension; cardiovascular disease[7]; urinary retention	Women[10]
	Imipramine				
	Lofepramine				
	Dosulepin[2]				
	Clomipramine[3]		OCD		
DRI	Bupropion	Smoking cessation		Risks of OD[5], seizures, anxiety, polypharmacy (↑interactions)	
SNRI	Venlafaxine	Treatment resistance; anxiety		Cardiac disease[7] (contraindicated)	
	Duloxetine	Urinary incontinence			
MRA	Agomelatine	Inconsistent use; ↓sleep		Liver disease (monitor LFTs)	

SSRI = selective serotonin reuptake inhibitor, SARI = serotonin antagonist and reuptake inhibitor, TCA = tricyclic antidepressant, DRI = dopamine reuptake inhibitor, SNRI = serotonin and noradrenaline reuptake inhibitor, NaSSA = noradrenaline and serotonin specific antidepressant; MRA = melatonin receptor agonists. 1 Escitalopram is the active enantiomer of citalopram. 2 Old name dothiepin 3 Also has serotonergic effects (hence efficacy in OCD) – only TCA with this effect. 4 Either concern about sexual dysfunction or experienced this on other antidepressants. 5 OD = overdose. 6 Can be oversedating initially and lead to intolerance – titrate up slowly and warn patient but reassure normally passes. 7 Associated with cardiac complications; monitor BP (± ECG) recommended. 8 Currently this is the best choice in most cases of child/adolescent depression due to less evidence of increasing suicidal ideation. 9 Has few drug interactions – particularly useful in the elderly. 10 Women poorly tolerate imipramine. 11 ↑risk of discontinuation syndrome. 12 ↑risk of suicidality.

How to prescribe

INSULIN

TYPES

Many exist, with differences in the timing of action onset **O**, peak **P** and duration **D**.

For acute use, e.g. sliding scales, inc perioperative:

- Soluble (aka normal/neutral) can be given **iv** (and **sc** as other types), e.g. Actrapid, Humulin S:

iv: **O/P** immediate, **D** 0.5 h. sc: **O** 0.5–1 h, **P** 2–4 h, **D** 6–8 h.

For maintenance use, i.e. normal chronic control (sc only):

- **Aspart** (NovoRapid), **lispro** (Humalog) or **glulisine** (▼ Apidra): recombinant human analogues. Rapid onset ⇒ ↑eating flexibility (can give immediately before meals; other types of sc insulin must be given 30 min before), ↓duration ⇒ fewer hypos (esp before meals). **O** 0.25 h, **P** 1–3 h, **D** 2–5 h. Usually given with intermediate- or long-acting insulin (= 'basal/bolus' regime).
- **Isophane:** intermediate-acting e.g. Humulin I, Insulatard or Insuman Basal, mostly given bd.
- **Glargine:** long-acting recombinant insulin with delayed and prolonged absorption from sc injection site ⇒ constant, more 'physiological' basal supply; mostly given od but can be split into bd dosing (e.g. Lantus).
- **Detemir:** long-acting analogue. Binds to albumin and has different action from that of glargine but similar advantages. Give od or bd (e.g. Levemir).

Biphasic insulins contain mixtures of intermediate- or long-acting insulin (e.g. isophane) with short-acting soluble insulin (e.g. aspart or lispro); e.g. Humalog Mix 25, Humulin M3, Insuman Comb 15, Insuman Comb 25, Novomix 30. Usually given bd (sometimes od).
  Short-acting insulins can also be given by continuous sc infusion, using a portable pump, which gives basal insulin with patient-activated boluses.

SLIDING SCALES

= Variable rate insulin ivi. For optimal blood glucose control in diabetics if (i) pre-operative/NBM, (ii) MI*/ACS*, (iii) severe concurrent illness (e.g. sepsis), (iv) DKA/HONK: for DKA see p. 253 (fixed rate ivi recommended rather than sliding scale, but this has yet to be implemented universally; follow local protocols).

Example of how to write an insulin sliding scale on a drug chart

DATE/ TIME	INFUSION FLUID	VOL- UME	ADDITIVES IF ANY DRUG AND DOSE	RATE OF ADMIN	DURA- TION	DR'S SIGNATURE	TIME START- ED	TIME COM- PLETED	SET UP BY SIG- NATURE	BATCH No.
08/01	Normal saline	50 ml	ACTRAPID 50 units	As below		TN				
08/01	Glucose saline	1 litre								
		CBG (= BM)	INSULIN ivi (ml/h)							
		0–4	0.5 (+ call Dr if CBG <2.5)							
		4.1–7	1							
		7.1–9	2							
		9.1–11	3							
		11.1–13	4							
		≥13.1	6							
Always run glucose saline (4% glucose + 0.18% saline) ivi at 125 ml per hour if CBG (BM) <1S.										

Figure 6 Drug chart, showing slide scale.

These are average requirements and ∴ only a suggested *initial* regimen: requirements will vary widely between individuals and within an individual over time (esp with intercurrent illness, e.g. infections). Regular review and adjustment is essential – see below. Use your hospital's protocols where possible.

Important points

- Carefully consider need for starting a sliding scale if patient eating/drinking normally and there is no other compelling indication; a poorly managed sliding scale ⇒ fluctuating glucose and ↑length of admission.
- ☠ When prescribing any insulin, never abbreviate the word 'units' to 'U' ('U' can be mistaken for 'O' leading to ten-fold dosing error' ☠.
- Check cannula working before adjusting sliding scale (if not working could be why BG not improving/↓ing). prn insulin is not recommended due to risk of hypoglycaemia.
- Always give 5% glucose or glucose saline (4% glucose with 0.18% saline, or 5% glucose with 0.45% saline and 0.15% KCl) ivi at 125 ml/h when CBG <15. If RF or mild HF give 5% glucose ivi at a slower rate. If severe HF give 10% glucose (preferably via central line) at 60–70 ml/h. KCl content should be adjusted according to individual needs (see pp. 224).
- State clearly to nursing staff the frequency with which CBGs are required: very sick patients need CBGs every 0.5–1 h and ideally regular laboratory BG readings (more accurate). If not very sick and CBGs stable (e.g. pre-operative), 2–4 hrly usually suffices.
- Stop oral hypoglycaemics and adjust for residual effects they may be having. Remember to reintroduce before stopping sliding scale!

*NB: glucose = dextrose. Low-strength glucose solutions used to be called dextrose solutions; this is now being phased out.

Amount of insulin: initial doses and adjustment

Prescribe 50 units of soluble insulin (Actrapid or Humulin S) in 50 ml normal (0.9% NaCl) saline to run via a syringe driver according to one of the regimens (A, B, C, D) below:

Before being attached to the patient: it is essential that intravenous line is primed and then flushed with 5 ml of the solution (as the plastic tubing adsorbs insulin) ∴ remaining volume will be 45 ml.

1 Start with regimen A, unless severe insulin resistance (i.e. normally takes ≥100 units sc insulin/day), in which case start with B.

2 If BG >10 (or >7 during acute MI, where target BG even lower) for 3 consecutive hourly tests and is ↑ing (or ↓ing by <25% in the past hour), step up to next sliding scale (i.e. if on A, step up to B; if on B, step up to C, etc).

3 If BG <3.5 mmol/l, step down to next scale (i.e. if on B, step down to A; if on C, step down to B, etc).

Coming off a sliding scale

Consider once eating/drinking normally and CBGs normal/stable:

- If post-DKA, change back only if blood free of ketones and pH back to normal.
- If postoperative and no reason to suppose change in needs (i.e. no infection), go straight back to pre-operative regimen.
- Avoid hypos by continuing ivi until 1st sc dose starts to work (usually 10–30 min). Always change from iv to sc before a meal.

CBG(= BM)	Insulin ivi (units/h)			
	Regime A	Regime B	Regime C**	Regime D**
0.0–4.0*	0.5	0.5	0.5	0.5
4.1–7.0	1	2	3	4
7.1–9.0	2	4	6	8
9.1–11.0	3	6	9	12
11.1–13.0	4	8	12	16
>13.0	6	12	18	24

*Stop ivi for 15 min if severe hypoglycaemia (CBG <2.5 or symptoms) and give Rx as on p. 256. Otherwise treat more gently with 5–10% glucose ivi and maintain insulin infusion (esp if DKA).
**Rarely needed; used mostly for patients with severe insulin resistance (i.e. on more than 100 units insulin/day before admission).
Reproduced with permission from Professor S Kumar, Dr A Rahim and Dr P Dyer, Endocrinology Department, University of Warwick Medical School.

The following is only a guide to how to start sc regimens (always consult your hospital's diabetes team if unsure):

1   Calculate daily requirements by doubling the number of units used in the past 12 h from the sliding scale. Note what fluids were given during this period.

2   Start qds sc regimen. If patient is well and CBGs very stable, this step may be omitted (i.e. go straight to a bd regimen). Give 1/3 of total daily dose at 10 pm (as intermediate, e.g. isophane, or long acting, e.g. glargine or determir, insulin) and give remaining 2/3 (as short-acting soluble insulin) divided equally between pre-breakfast, pre-lunch and pre-evening meal doses.

3   Start bd sc regimen: give 60% of daily dose pre-breakfast and the remaining 40% pre-evening meal, both doses as biphasic 30/70 insulin (e.g. Humulin M3). Enquire about previous insulin regimens and control.

PRE-OPERATIVE GUIDELINES: GENERAL POINTS (FOR ALL PATIENTS)

Local protocols should be used if they exist, otherwise a sensible way to progress would be to:

• Ensure patient 1st on operating list and fast from midnight*.
• Stop all long-acting insulins the night before the operation.
• Withhold all DM medications for morning of operation.
• Prescribe 5 or 10% glucose ivi in case of hypoglycaemia.
• Proceed as per table below**.

*If pm-only list, give light breakfast and normal morning medications (but no intermediate/long acting insulins), monitor CBG 1–2-hrly. Start sliding scale/GIK at 11 am (unless well controlled type II) or if CBGs uncontrolled.

 **If sliding scale required, NHS Diabetes guideline (Management of adults with diabetes undergoing surgery and elective procedures, April 2011) recommends that 1st choice fluid for ivi is 0.45% saline with 5% glucose and either 0.15% or 0.3% KCl.

Type of surgery	Type II (control good)	Type II (control poor/fasting glucose > 10) or Type 1
	Monitor CBGs 2-hrly	Monitor CBGs 1-hrly
Minor: expect to eat normally the same day	After operation give normal medications ASAP with a meal (sliding scale not usually required)	Start sliding scale/GIK at 10 pm the night before op. Give normal medications and meal ASAP after operation
Major/GI: not expected to eat the same day	Start sliding scale/GIK if CBGs not controlled**. Convert back to normal medications once CBGs stable and eating/drinking normally	Start sliding scale/GIK at 10 pm the night before operation. Convert back to normal medications once CBGs stable and eating/drinking normally

**Uncontrolled CBGs = single reading >15 or consistently >10.

ANTICOAGULANTS

WARFARIN

> Consult your local anticoagulant service if unsure about indications, doses or interactions. Refer as early before discharge as practicable so outpatient monitoring is arranged in time.

Basics
Oral anticoagulant for long-term Rx/Px of TE: loading (see below) usually takes several days and is initially prothrombotic, so heparin (LMWH), which is effective immediately, is used as short-term cover until therapeutic levels are achieved.

Monitoring
Via INR = ratio of patient's PT (prothrombin time) to a control raised to the power of a variable dependent on exact reagents used in each lab. A target INR is set at the start of Rx, according to indication (see below); variations of ±0.5 are acceptable.

BCSH guidelines for target INRs. Adapted with permission from *British Journal of Haematology* 2011; **154**(3): 311–24.

Indication	Target INR ($\pm$ 0.5)
DVT/PE[1]	2.5
Thrombophilia (if symptomatic)[2]	2.5
Paroxysmal nocturnal haemoglobinuria (PNH)[3]	2.5
AF[4] (or other causes of cardiac emboli[5])	2.5
Bioprosthetic heart valves[6]	2.5
Mechanical heart valves[7]	3.5

1 Treat for =6 weeks if calf vein thrombosis, for =3 months if provoked proximal (peroneal or above) DVT/PE, for =6 months or lifelong if diopathic venous TE or permanent risk factors. If recurrent DVT/PE whilst on therapeutic Rx, target INR = 3.5. Discuss all other than 1st presentation with anticoagulant service.

2 Arterial thrombosis in antiphospholipid syndrome is exception with target INR 3.5.

3 Paroxysmal nocturnal haemoglobinuria (PNH); only under guidance of consultant haematologist.

4 Maintain INR >2.0 for 3 weeks before and 4 weeks after elective DC cardioversion.

5 Dilated cardiomyopathy, mural thrombus post-MI or rheumatic value disease.

6 Only for first 3–6 months post value insertion at discretion of each centre.

7 For new generation aortic values INR target 3.0.

Although not yet in the BCSH guidelines, a target INR of 2.5 is widely agreed for nephrotic syndrome (generally once albumin <20 g/l).

Starting Rx (for acute thrombosis)

Check INR before 1st dose and every day for 4 days, then assess stability of INR and adjust accordingly. If on LMWH, do not stop until 2 days after therapeutic INR achieved.

For loading regimens, where possible use your hospital's own guidelines, since these often vary. Otherwise, it is sensible to use the BCSH guidelines:

Warfarin loading regimen. Adapted with permission of BMJ group from Fennerty A, *et al. BMJ* 1984; **288**: 1268–1270.

Day 1		Day 2		Day 3		Day 4	
INR	Dose (mg)	INR	Dose (mg)	INR	Dose (mg)	INR	Dose* (mg)
<1.4	10	<1.8	10	<2.0	10	<1.4	>8
		1.8	1	2.0–2.1	5	1.4	8
		>1.8	0.5	2.2–2.3	4.5	1.5	7.5
				2.4–2.5	4	1.6–1.7	7
				2.6–2.7	3.5	1.8	6.5
				2.8–2.9	3	1.9	6
				3.0–3.1	2.5	2.0–2.1	5.5
				3.2–3.3	2	2.2–2.3	5
				3.4	1.5	2.4–2.6	4.5
				3.5	1	2.7–3.0	4
				3.6–4.0	0.5	3.1–3.5	3.5
				>4.0	0	3.6–4.0	3
						4.1–4.5	Miss 1 day then 2 mg
						>4.5	Miss 2 days then 1 mg

*Predicted maintenance dose.

Situations when doses (especially loading) may need review
↓**doses if:** age >80 yrs, LF, HF, post-op, poor nutrition, ↑baseline INR or taking drugs that potentiate warfarin (check for **W+** symbols in this book) including almost all antibiotics.
↑**doses if:** taking drugs that inhibit warfarin (check for **W−** symbols in this book).
Herbal remedies/non-prescription drugs: can have significant interactions – always ask patients directly if taking any, as they may not realise the importance (e.g. glucosamine can ↑INR). Check each one with your hospital's drug information office for significance.

> **Alcohol and diet:** can affect dosing, especially if intake varies – the goalposts will move for an individual's therapeutic range.
> *It is a common misconception that BMI influences response.*

NB: slow loading with 3–5 mg for 5–7 days achieves therapeutic levels with less overshoot and may be preferable for outpatient initiation in atrial fibrillation. (BCSH guidelines 3rd edition 2005 update www.bcshguidelines.com.)

If interrupting warfarin (e.g. before operation/procedure), assess thrombotic risk and use bridging anticoagulation with LMWH as necessary; do not reload post-op as above, but restart at usual dose +50% for 2 days, then return to usual dose *if no contraindications* (e.g. bleeding/taking **W**+ drugs).

> Make small infrequent dose changes unless INR dangerously high or low. 'Steering a supertanker' is a good analogy; there is often significant delay between dose changes and their fx.

Warfarin and surgery

Warfarin is often stopped 4–5 days ahead of surgery and other invasive procedures ($\pm$ heparin cover until day of procedure). Exact protocol depends on procedure involved and risks of bleeding versus thrombosis: get senior advice from team doing the procedure and haematologists if at all unsure.

Warfarin and pregnancy

Warfarin is contraindicated in early pregnancy (teratogenic during weeks 6–12). Women of childbearing age must be counselled by a specialist prior to planning pregnancy (inc informed to do pregnancy test whenever a period is >2 days late) and any woman who is pregnant and on warfarin must be converted immediately to LMWH under specialist guidance.

> *Overtreatment/poisoning*
> *Seek expert help from haematology on-call* as xs vitamin K can make
> re-anticoagulation difficult, as fx can last for weeks ∴ ⇒ ↑risk from
> condition that warfarin was started for.

Recommendations for Mx of excess warfarin (BCSH guidelines). Adapted with
permission from *British Journal of Haematology* 2011; **154**(3): 311–24.

INR	Action
3.0–6.0 if target 2.5 (4.0–6.0 if target 3.5)	↓dose or stop warfarin; restart when INR <5.0
6.0–8.0 and no/minor bleeding	Stop warfarin; restart when INR <5.0
>8.0 and no/minor bleeding	Stop warfarin; restart when INR <5.0
	If other bleeding risks (e.g. age > 70 yrs, Hx of bleeding complications or liver disease) give phytomenadione (vit K_1) 0.5mg* iv or 5mg po
Major bleeding, e.g. ↓ing Hb or cardiodynamic instability	Stop warfarin Phytomenadione (vit K_1) 5 or 10mg iv, repeating 24h later if necessary Prothrombin complex concentrate 30–50 units/kg not exceeding 3000 units (if unavailable give FFP** 15ml/kg)

*Since the publication of the BCSH guidelines some clinicians advise larger doses of iv vit K, e.g. 2mg

**Although not stated in the BCSH guidelines it should be noted that FFP is not fully effective at warfarin reversal.

DABIGATRAN

Dabigatran etexilate (▼ Pradaxa), a direct thrombin inhibitor, is a
new oral anticoagulant licensed for once-daily administration for
extended thromboprophylaxis after elective total knee or hip replacement[NICE]. It doesn't require monitoring of anticoagulant fx, and has
fewer drug–food interactions than warfarin. NB: Caution if LF or RF.

HEPARIN

For immediate and short-term Rx/Px of TE. Two major types: low-molecular-weight heparins (LMWHs) and unfractionated heparin.

LMWHs

Given sc. ↑convenience (↓monitoring, can give to outpatients). ↓incidence of HIT* and osteoporosis cf unfractionated heparin means now preferred for most indications (esp MI/ACS, DVT/PE Rx and pre-cardioversion of AF). Dalteparin (Fragmin), enoxaparin (Clexane) and tinzaparin (Innohep) are the most commonly used; each hospital tends to use one in particular; ask nurses which one they stock or call pharmacy. Prophylaxis does not need monitoring but do not use for >7–10 days if creatinine >150.

Monitoring of treatment with LMWH

Via peak anti-Xa assay: usually necessary only if renal impairment (i.e. creatinine >150), pregnancy or at extremes of Wt (i.e. <45 kg or >100 kg). Take sample 3–4 h post dose.

> *HIT* = heparin-induced thrombocytopenia*
> Much more common with unfractionated heparin but can occur with all heparins. Watch for ↓ing platelet count. Get senior help if concerned. Discuss investigation and Mx with haematologist. If HIT confirmed, stop heparin immediately – danaparoid (Orgaran) or lepirudin (Refludan) may be substituted.

Unfractionated heparin

Given iv*: quickly reversible (immediately if protamine given; see p. 214), which makes it useful in settings where desired amount of anticoagulation may change rapidly, e.g. perioperatively, if patient at ↑risk of bleeding, or if using extracorporeal circuits such as cardio-pulmonary bypass and haemodialysis. Can also be used with recombinant fibrinolytics in AMI. Due to difficulty keeping in therapeutic range, LMWH increasingly preferred where possible – discuss with senior if contemplating use.

*Can be given sc (only for Px), but now largely replaced by LMWH.

Monitoring

Via APTT ratio (= **A**ctivated **P**artial **T**hromboplastin **T**ime of patient plasma divided by that of control plasma). Results can (rarely) be given as patient's exact APTT: the normal range is 35–45 sec. You then need to calculate the ratio: take the middle of the normal range for your lab (e.g. 40 sec) for your calculations. *Target ratio is commonly 1.5–2.5*, but this can vary: check your hospital's protocol and aim for the middle of range. NB: there is no national (let alone international) consensus on methods of measuring APTT, so results are not yet standardised.

Starting iv treatment

1 *Load with 5000** units as iv bolus*: prescribed on the 'once-only' section of the drug chart (give 10 000** units if severe PE).

2 Set up ivi at 15–25 units/kg/h: usually = 1000–2000 units/h. A sensible starting rate is 1500 units/h, which can be achieved by adding 25 000 units of heparin to 48 ml of normal saline to make 50 ml of solution (500 units/ml), which runs at 3 ml/h via a syringe driver. This can be written up as follows:

DATE/ TIME	INFUSION FLUID	VOLUME	ADDITIVES IF ANY DRUG AND DOSE	RATE OF ADMIN	DURA-TION	DR'S SIGNATURE	TIME START-ED	TIME COM-PLETED	SET UP BY SIG-NATURE	BATCH No.
08/01	*Normal saline*	*50 ml*	*HEPARIN 25,000 units*			*TN*				
	run at 3 ml per hour as ivi									

Figure 7 Drug chart showing how to write up heparin infusion.

> *NB*
> Dosing for co-therapy with fibrinolytics (according to ESC guidelines) is slightly different; see p. 215.

Check APTT ratio after 6 h, then 6–10 h until stable, and then daily at a minimum, adjusting to the following regimen:

This regimen is based on APTT *ratio* therapeutic range of 1.5–2.5. *Don't take sample from drip arm* (unless from site distal to ivi).

APTT ratio	Action
<1.2	Give 5000-unit bolus iv and ↑ivi by 200–250 units/h
1.2–1.5	Give 2500-unit bolus iv and ↑ivi by 100–150 units/h
1.5–2.5	No change
2.5–3.0	↓ivi by 100–150 units/h
>3.0	Stop ivi for 1h then restart ivi, ↓ing by 200–250 units/h

Adjustments are safest made by writing a fresh ivi prescription at a different strength, but the same effect can also be achieved by calculating the appropriate rate change to the original prescription.

Variable rate of ivi (for fixed prescription of 25 000 units heparin in 50 ml saline):

Desired heparin ivi rate (units/h)	Rate of ivi (ml/h)	Desired heparin ivi rate (units/h)	Rate of ivi (ml/h)
1000	2.0	1500	3.0
1050	2.1	1550	3.1
1100	2.2	1600	3.2
1150	2.3	1650	3.3
1200	2.4	1700	3.4
1250	2.5	1750	3.5
1300	2.6	1800	3.6
1350	2.7	1850	3.7
1400	2.8	1900	3.8
1450	2.9	1950	3.9

Overtreatment/poisoning (all heparins)

If significant bleeding, stop heparin and observe: iv heparin has short $t_{1/2}$ (30 min–2 h), so fx wear off quickly. If bleeding continues or is life-threatening, consider iv protamine (1 mg per 80–100 units of heparin to be neutralised as ivi over 10 min. ↓doses if giving >15 min after heparin stopped). NB: protamine is less effective against LMWH, and repeat administration may be required.

Seek expert help from haematology on-call if in any doubt!

▼ FONDAPARINUX

A new parenteral anticoagulant (synthetic pentasaccharide). Licensed for use in Rx of VTE and MI/ACS and Px of VTE in medical patients and patients undergoing orthopaedic or abdominal surgery. Monitoring is not necessary. Useful for Px of VTE for patients with history of HIT* or allergy to heparin. See BNF/SPC for dosing. NB: Caution if RF or LF.

THROMBOLYSIS

Thrombolysis is indicated for ischaemic complications of TE. Fibrinolytic drugs activate plasminogen to form plasmin that degrades fibrin. They are most commonly used for acute MI (though more commonly now patients undergo primary angioplasty), ischaemic stroke or PE, but can also be used for other arterial (or venous) TE such as DVT, central retinal venous (or arterial) thrombosis, acute arterial TE or for clearing clotted catheters/cannulas. Most fibrinolytics are only licensed for some of these indications[BNF]. Common side effects are bleeding (mostly mild and at iv sites; if severe or suspect cerebral bleed occurring, stop ivi and get senior help), N&V, ↓BP (improves if transiently ↓rate of ivi and raise legs). Serious reperfusion arrhythmias and mild hypersensitivity (inc uveitis) can also occur. Anaphylaxis and GBS occur rarely.

General guidance on thrombolysis for MI and stroke are as follows but always check your local protocol:

ACUTE MI; see pp. 240 for other steps in management

Indications

(From Resuscitation Council (UK) guidelines 2010):

- Onset of (cardiac) chest pain <12 h + Hx compatible with MI + one of:

- ST elevation ≥ 2 mV ($= 2$ small squares) in ≥ 2 adjacent chest leads
- ST elevation > 1 mV ($= 1$ small square) in > 2 limb leads
- new LBBB: must assume it is new if cannot prove is old
- Onset of chest pain 12–24 h ago and evidence of an evolving infarct, e.g. ongoing chest pain or worsening ECG changes.

Note:

- Primary PCI is 1st line treatment for all patients presenting with acute MI if available.
- Posterior infarcts are also widely considered to be an indication for primary PCI or thrombolysis. Diagnosis can be hard (look for ST depression + dominant R wave in V1–3); get cardiology advice if suspicious.
- Treatment needs to be started ASAP as 'time = myocardium' and 'door to needle time' is important.

☠ **Contraindications** ☠
From ESC guidelines 2008 (with permission from *European Heart Journal* 2008; **29**: 2909–2945). Local guidelines/checklists often exist and should be used if available: consult cardiology $\pm$ haematology on-call if in any doubt.

Absolute
- Haemorrhagic stroke or stroke of unknown origin at any time
- Ischaemic stroke in preceding 6 months
- CNS trauma or neoplasms
- Major trauma/surgery/head injury in preceding 3 weeks
- GI bleeding within the last month
- Known bleeding disorder
- Aortic dissection
- Non-compressible punctures (e.g. liver biopsy, lumbar puncture).

Relative
- TIA in past 6 months
- Oral anticoagulant therapy

- Pregnancy or within 1-wk post partum
- Refractory resuscitation
- Refractory hypertension (systolic >180 mmHg and/or diastolic >110 mmHg)
- Advanced liver disease
- Infective endocarditis
- Active peptic ulcer.

CHOICE OF AGENT

Always use your hospital's protocol if one exists – contact CCU, A&E or look on your hospital intranet for details.

Choose between streptokinase and a recombinant thrombolytic such as alteplase, reteplase or tenecteplase (each hospital tends to stock one in particular); see individual drug entries in common drugs section for dosing regimens.

NICE guidance recommends that, in hospitals, the choice of agent should take account of:

- 'The likely balance of benefit and harm (e.g. stroke) to which each of the thrombolytic agents would expose the individual patient.' Recombinant forms (compared with streptokinase) are probably more efficacious and have ↓incidence of allergic reactions, CCF and bleeding other than stroke. However they have ↑incidence of haemorrhagic stroke.
- 'Current UK clinical practice, in which it is accepted that patients who have previously received streptokinase should not be treated with it again.' Streptokinase is less effective and more likely to cause allergic reaction after first administration (due to Ab production). Don't give if patient has been given it in the past.
- 'The hospital's arrangements for reducing delays in the administration of thrombolysis.' Some agents are quicker to set up and administer and this can reduce 'door to needle times'.

> *Heparin co-therapy*
> *Recombinant* forms always need concurrent iv heparin for 24–48 h
> (this does not usually apply for *streptokinase*). Use your hospital's
> A&E/CCU protocol if one exists. Otherwise use *ESC guidelines:*
> 60 units/kg (max 4000 units) iv bolus, then ivi at 12 units/kg/h for
> 24–48 h (max 1000 units/h). Monitor APTT at 3, 6, 12, 24 and 48 h,
> with target APTT ($\neq$ APTT ↑*ratio*!) of 50–70 sec. NB: this is different
> from 'standard' iv heparin regimens (see p. 212).

ACUTE ISCHAEMIC STROKE see algorithm on inside back
cover for other steps in management.

Currently only alteplase is licensed for this indication and only if given
≤3 h from symptom onset (although ECASS-III trial shows evidence
of benefit ≤4.5 h).

- Act quickly: 5% ↓ in efficacy per 5 min delay. Aim for 'door to
  needle' time of 30 min.
- Determine **exact** time of onset of 1st symptoms. If not clear, the last
  time patient was known to be normal should be used.
- Ensure glucose normal (e.g. check CBG).

Haemorrhagic stroke (or ↑risk of) needs to be excluded; perform brain
imaging immediately if any of the following apply[NICE]:

- Indications for thrombolysis (see below) or early anticoagulation
  treatment
- On anticoagulant treatment
- Known bleeding tendency
- ↓GCS (<13)
- Unexplained progressive or fluctuating symptoms
- Papilloedema, neck stiffness or fever
- Severe headache at onset of stroke symptoms.

Indications and contraindications vary according to centre and
research into risk/benefit is ongoing; always ensure you check your

local protocol. Most centres currently use similar criteria to those shown on the next page.

NB: Consent (where possible) according to latest evidence: e.g. 1:8 chance of ↑improvement and 1:30 chance of symptomatic bleed.

When all of the above are satisfied give alteplase: total dose = 0.9 mg/kg (maximum 90 mg). 10% given as iv bolus over 2 min, remaining 90% given over 60 min via iv pump. Dissolve in water for injections to a concentration of 1 mg/ml or 2 mg/ml.

Indications	Contraindications
Clinical signs of acute stroke	Rapidly improving or minor symptoms
Clear time of onset	Stroke or serious head injury in last 3 months
Treatment within 3 h of onset	Past history of intracranial haemorrhage
Haemorrhage excluded on brain imaging	Recent major surgery, GI bleed, etc.
Age 18–80 yrs**	BP > 185/110mmHg*
Some centres use NIHSS to define	INR > 1.6 or other clotting disorder
Suitable severity (e.g. score of 5–25, but can vary)	Infarction of >1/3 MCA territory seen on CT
	Fit at onset

*If ↑BP is a contraindication can ↓BP with labetalol or GTN; get senior advice.

**Often given to older patients.

Post-thrombolysis management

- Bed rest for 24 h (flat bed recommended initially)
- Treat ↓O₂/↓glucose if present
- ↓glucose if >8 mmol/l
- Observations: every 15 min for 2 h, every 30 min for 6 h, then hrly
- No antiplatelet therapy for 24 h. Avoid cannulas, NGTs and ivis
- If BP >180/105 mmHg consider labetalol 10 mg iv over 1–2 min, then infusion at 2–8 mg/min
- If intracranial haemorrhage occurs, consider 5–10 units cryo-precipitate (± platelets ± FFP) and seek neurosurgical opinion.

CONTROLLED DRUGS

In the UK special 'Prescription requirements' apply to 'schedule' 1, 2 or 3 drugs only, the most likely of which to be prescribed by junior doctors are morphine, diamorphine, fentanyl, methadone, oxycodone (and less commonly buprenorphine or pethidine). The following must be written 'so as to be indelible, e.g. written by hand, typed or computer generated' (NB: *this is a recent change from previously having to be written by hand – only the signature now needs to be handwritten*):

- Date
- The patient's full name and address and, where appropriate, age
- Drug name plus its form* (and, where appropriate, strength)
- Dosing regimen (NB: the directions 'take one as directed' constitutes a dose but 'as directed' does not)
- Total amount of drug to be dispensed *in words and figures* (e.g. for morphine 5 mg qds for one week (5 mg × 4 times a day × 7 days = 140) write: '140 milligrams = one hundred and forty milligrams')
- Prescriber's address must be specified (should already be on prescription form, e.g. hospital address).

*Omitting the form (e.g. tablet/liquid/patch) is a common reason for an invalid prescription. It is often assumed to be obvious from the prescription (e.g. fentanyl as a patch or Oramorph as a liquid), but it still has to be written even if only one form exists.

  These requirements *don't* apply to temazepam (despite being schedule 3), schedule 4 drugs (e.g. benzodiazepines) and schedule 5 drugs (such as codeine, dihydrocodeine/DF118 and tramadol). For full details on controlled drug guidance in the UK see www.dh.gov.uk/controlleddrugs.

Miscellaneous

INTRAVENOUS FLUIDS

CRYSTALLOIDS

Isotonic: used mostly for maintenance (replacement) regimens:

- *Normal (0.9%) saline:* 1 litre contains 154 mmol Na^+. Use as default maintenance fluid in all situations unless local protocol dictates otherwise. Caution in $\uparrow Na^+$ and liver dysfunction.
- *5% glucose*:* 1 litre contains 278 mmol ($= 50$ g) glucose, which is rapidly taken up by cells and included only to make the fluid isotonic (calories are minimal, at 200 kcal). Used as method of giving pure H_2O and as ivi with insulin sliding scales (see p. 203). NB: commonest cause of $\downarrow Na^+$ in hospital is overuse of 5% glucose as fluid replacement.
- *Glucose* saline:* 1 litre contains mixture of NaCl (30 mmol Na^+) and glucose (4% $= 222$ mmol). Useful as contains correct proportions of constituents (excluding KCl, which can be added to each bag) for average daily requirements (see below). Suboptimal long term, as does not account for individual patient needs (esp if these are far from average). Also used as ivi in insulin sliding scales (see p. 203).
- *Hartmann's solution:* compound sodium lactate, used in surgery/trauma (also 1 litre contains 5 mmol K^+). Avoid if RF.

Non-isotonic: used less commonly; only for use in specialist/emergency situations by those accustomed to their use:

- *Hypertonic (5%) saline:* 1 litre contains 856 mmol Na^+; given mostly for severe hyponatraemia. ☠ Seek specialist help first ☠.
- *Hypotonic (0.45%) saline:* for severe $\uparrow Na^+$ (e.g. HONK).
- *10% and 20% glucose*:* for mild/moderate hypoglycaemia.
- *50% glucose*:* for severe hypoglycaemia (see p. 256) and if insulin being used to lower K^+ (see p. 258).
- *Sodium bicarbonate (1.26% or move rarely 1.4%):* useful replacement for 0.9% saline if $\downarrow pH$ or $\uparrow K^+$ which often coexist. Not isotonic so caution re: salt load and accompanying fluid retention. ☠ Seek specialist help from nephrologists/others accustomed to its use ☠.

*NB: glucose = dextrose. Low-strength glucose solutions used to be called dextrose solutions; this is now being phased out.

COLLOIDS (= plasma substitutes/expanders)

- Gelofusine: gelatin-based and used in resuscitation of shock (non-cardiogenic). NB: the electrolyte contents are often overlooked: 1 litre Gelofusine has 154 mmol Na^+.
- *Blood/packed cells:* helpful to ↑/maintain plasma oncotic pressure.

STANDARD DAILY REQUIREMENTS

= 3 litres H_2O, 40–70 mmol K^+, 100–150 mmol Na^+.

If no oral intake (preoperative, ↓GCS, unsafe swallow, post-CVA, etc), this can be provided as follows:

DATE	INFUSION FLUID	VOL-UME	ADDITIVES IF ANY DRUG AND DOSE	RATE OF ADMIN	DURA-TION	DR'S SIGNATURE	TIME START-ED	TIME COM-PLETED	SET UP BY SIG-NATURE	BATCH No.
08/01	5% Glucose	1 litre	20 mmol KCl		8h	TN				
08/01	Normal saline	1 litre			8h	TN				
08/01	5% Glucose	1 litre	20 mmol KCl		8h	TN				

Figure 8 Drug chart showing how to write up intravenous fluids.

This '2 sweet (5% glucose), 1 sour (0.9% saline)' regimen is commonly used in fit pre-operative patients. If in any doubt, normal (0.9%) saline is generally safest unless liver failure (see below) or if Na^+ outside normal range (↓ or ↑). Always get senior help if unsure: incorrect fluids can be as dangerous as any other drug.

Individual requirements may differ substantially according to:

- Body habitus, age, residual oral intake, if on multiple iv drugs (which are sometimes given with significant amounts of fluid).
- Insensible losses (normally about 1 litre/day). ↑skin losses if fever or burns. ↑lung losses in hyperventilation or inhalation burns.

- GI losses (normally about 0.2 litre/day). Any vomiting ($\uparrow Cl^-$ content) or diarrhoea ($\uparrow K^+$ content) must be taken into account as well as less obvious causes, e.g. ileus, fistulae.
- Fluid compartment shifts, esp vasodilation if sepsis/anaphylaxis.

All the above points seem obvious but are easy to forget!

K^+ CONSIDERATIONS

Do not give >10 mmol/h unless K^+ dangerously low, when it can be given quicker (see p. 259). Surgical patients often need less K^+ in 1st 24 h post-op, as K^+ is released by cell death ($\therefore$ proportional to extent of surgery).

IMPORTANT POINTS

- Take extreme care if major organ failure:
  - *Heart failure:* heart can quickly become 'overloaded' and $\Rightarrow$ acute LVF. Even if not currently in HF, beware if predisposed (e.g. Hx of HF or IHD).
  - *Renal failure:* unless pre-renal cause (e.g. hypovolaemia), do not give more fluid than residual renal function can deal with. Seek help from renal team if at all concerned; good fluid Mx greatly influences outcomes in this group. Only use saline unless specialist advice taken.
  - *Liver failure:* often preferable to use 5% glucose. Serum Na^+ may be $\downarrow$d, but total body Na^+ is often $\uparrow$d. Any saline will work its way into the wrong compartment (e.g. peritoneal fluid $\therefore$ $\uparrow$ing ascites) but may be essential to ensure renal perfusion (RF often coexists).
- If in doubt, give 'fluid challenges': small volumes (normally 200–500 ml) of fluid over short periods of time, to see whether clinical response to BP, urine output or left ventricular function is beneficial or detrimental before committing to longer-term fluid strategy.
- In general, encourage oral fluids: homeostasis (if normal) is safer, less expensive and less consuming of doctor/nurse time than iv fluids. Beware if $\downarrow$swallow, fluid overload (esp if HF or RF), pre-/post-operative or if homeostasis disorders (esp SIADH).

- Check the following before prescribing any iv fluids:
  - *Clinical markers of hydration:* skin turgor/temperature, mucous membranes, JVP, peripheral oedema, pulmonary oedema. Often overlooked and very useful!
  - *Recent input and output:* if at all concerned, ask nurses for strict fluid balance chart. However, on a busy ward this is difficult to achieve so daily weights often most informative.
  - Recent U&Es, esp K^+.

It can be difficult to elicit all this information under time pressure. The trick is to know when to take extreme care. Be particularly careful if you do not know the patient when on call, and be wary when asked to 'just write up another bag' without reviewing the patient. Often, you will be asked to prescribe fluids when no longer necessary or even when they may be harmful. To save time for those on call (and to ↑ the chances of your patients getting appropriate fluids), leave clear instructions with the nurses and on the drug chart for as long as can be sensibly predicted (esp over weekends/long holidays).

STEROIDS

CORTICOSTEROIDS

The most commonly used systemic drugs are:

Drug	Equivalent dose	Main uses
Prednisolone	5 mg	Acute asthma/COPD, rheumatoid arthritis (po)
Methylprednisolone	4 mg	Acute flares rheumatoid arthritis/MS (iv)
Dexamethasone	750 microgram	↑ICP, CAH, Dx Cushing's (iv/po)
Hydrocortisone	20 mg	Acute asthma/COPD (iv)

Glucocorticoid fx predominate; mineralocorticoid fx for these are all mild apart from hydrocortisone (has moderate fx) and dexamethasone (has minimal fx ∴ used when H_2O and Na^+ retention are particularly undesirable, e.g. ↑ICP).

Side effects = Cushing's syndrome!

- *Metabolic*: Na^+/fluid retention*, hyperlipoproteinaemia, leukocytosis, negative K^+/Ca^{2+}/nitrogen balance, generalised fluid/electrolyte abnormalities.
- *Endocrine*: hyperglycaemia/↓GTT (can ⇒ DM), adrenal suppression.
  - *Fat**: truncal obesity, moon face, interscapular ('buffalo hump') and suprascapular fat pads.
  - *Skin*: hirsutism, bruising/purpura, acne, striae, ↓healing, telangiectasia, thinning.
  - *Other*: impotence, menstrual irregularities/amenorrhoea, ↓growth (children), ↑appetite*.
- *GI*: pancreatitis, peptic/oesophageal ulcers: give PPI if on ↑doses.
- *Cardiac*: HTN, CCF, myocardial rupture post-MI, TE.
- *Musculoskeletal*: proximal myopathy, osteoporosis, fractures (can ⇒ avascular necrosis).
- *Neurological*: ↑epilepsy, ↑ICP/papilloedema (esp children on withdrawal of corticosteroids).
- *Ψ*: mood Δs (↑ or ↓), psychosis (esp at ↑doses), dependence.
- *Ocular*: cataracts, glaucoma, corneal/scleral thinning.
- *Infections*: ↑susceptibility, ↑speed (↑severity at presentation), TB reactivation, ↑risk of chickenpox/shingles/measles.

> *SEs are dose-dependent*
> If patient is on high doses, make sure this is intentional: it is not rare in fluctuating (e.g. inflammatory) illnesses for patients to be left on high doses by mistake. Seek specialist advice if unsure. If on long term Rx consider giving Ca/vit D supplements/ bisphosphonate to ↓risk of osteoporosis and PPI to ↓risk of GI ulcer.

> **Cautions**
> Can mostly be worked out from the SEs. Caution should be taken if patient already has a condition that is a potential SE. Systemic corticosteroids are CI in systemic infections (w/o antibiotic cover). NB: avoid live vaccines. If never had chickenpox, avoid exposure.

Interactions

Apply to all systemic Rx. fx can be ↓d by rifampicin, carbamazepine, phenytoin and phenobarbital. fx can be ↑d by erythromycin, ketoconazole, itraconazole and ciclosporin (whose own fx are ↑d by methylprednisolone). ↑risk of ↓K^+ with amphotericin and digoxin.

Withdrawal effects

Acute adrenal insufficiency (= Addisonian crisis; ☠ can be fatal ☠ see p. 257): ↓BP, fever, myalgia, arthralgia, rhinitis, conjunctivitis, painful itchy nodules, ↓Wt. ∴ must withdraw slowly if patient has had >3 wks Rx (or a shorter course w/in 1 year of stopping long-term Rx), other causes of adrenal suppression, received high doses (>40 mg od prednisolone or equivalent), or repeat doses in evening, or repeat course. Also note intercurrent illness, trauma, surgery needs ↑doses and can precipitate relative withdrawal.

Steroid Rx card must be carried by all patients on prolonged Rx.

MINERALOCORTICOIDS e.g. fludrocortisone

Used for Addison's disease and acute adrenocortical deficiency (rarely needed for hypopituitarism). Can also be used for orthostatic/postural hypotension. Main SEs are H_2O/Na^+ retention.

SEDATION/SLEEPING TABLETS

ACUTE SEDATION/RAPID TRANQUILLISATION

For the acutely agitated, disturbed or violent patient (and for temporary sedation before unpleasant procedures).

Important points

- Organic causes (i.e. delirium) are commonest cause outside of Ψ wards: look for and treat sepsis, hypoxia, drug withdrawal (esp alcohol/opiates) and metabolic causes (esp hypoglycaemia).
- A well-lit calm room and reassurance can be all that is required.
- Oral medications should be tried first if possible.
- Obtain as much drug Hx as possible, esp of antipsychotics and benzodiazepines as influences selection of appropriate agent/dose.

There are two main choices: antipsychotics and benzodiazepines:
☺ good for/reasons to choose; ☹ bad for/reasons to not give.

Antipsychotics

- ☺ Taking benzodiazepines, elderly (use with caution, esp if ↑ risk of CVA), delirium (non-alcohol withdrawal), psychosis (e.g. hallucinations/delusions/schizophrenia).
- ☹ Antipsychotic-naive, alcohol withdrawal, cardiac disease, movement disorders (esp Parkinson's; de novo extrapyramidal fx are also common – see p. 236).
- *Haloperidol* 0.5–5 mg po (or im/iv if necessary). 1–2 mg is sensible starting dose for delirium in elderly. 5 mg is safe for acute psychosis in young adults. Maximum 18 mg im or 30 mg po in 24 h.
- If suspect *acute schizophrenia* use atypical antipsychotic as 1st-line[NICE], e.g. olanzapine 10 mg po (⇒ ↓SEs) – now also available im.

Benzodiazepines

- ☺ Alcohol withdrawal, anxiety.
- ☹ Respiratory disease (⇒ respiratory depression; care if COPD/asthma), elderly (⇒ falls and rarely paradoxical agitation/aggression but can use with caution/↓ doses).
- *Lorazepam* 0.5–1 mg po/im/iv (maximum 4 mg/24 h). Shorter-acting than diazepam ∴ better if hepatic impairment.
- *Diazepam* 2–5 mg po/iv (if iv preferably as Diazemuls) or 10–20 mg pr. Can ↑doses[SPC/BNF] esp if tolerance/much previous exposure to benzodiazepines.
- *Midazolam* 1.0–7.5 mg iv: titrate up slowly, according to response. Requires iv access and is used mostly for cooperative patients ahead of unpleasant procedures (less suitable for very agitated patients). Also wears off relatively quickly.

SLEEPING TABLETS

Try to avoid giving:

- For >2–4 wks (dependency common). Try reassurance/↑'sleep hygiene' (see www.rcpsych.ac.uk/mentalhealthinfoforall/problems/

sleepproblems/sleepingwell.aspx)/non-pharmacological measures
1st. Treat depression if 1° cause.

- At all if hepatic encephalopathy or ↓respiratory reserve (esp asthma/
COPD; NB: *hypoxia can also* ⇒ *restlessness and agitation!*).

Choose from:

1 **Benzodiazepines:** ↑the major inhibitory neurotransmitter GABA
via their own (benzodiazepine) receptor.

- *Temazepam* 10 mg nocte (can ↑to 20 mg).

Halve doses if LF (avoid if severe; consider oxazepam, or lorazepam
instead), RF or elderly.

2 **'Z'/Benzodiazepine-like drugs:** similarly ↑s GABA.

- *Zopiclone* 7.5 mg nocte
- *Zolpidem* 10 mg nocte
- *Zaleplon* 10 mg nocte.

Halve doses if LF (avoid if severe), RF or elderly.

3 **Sedating antihistamines:** are a good alternative: ⇒ ↓respiratory
depression/addiction but ↑hangover drowsiness; effectiveness may
↓ after several days of Rx ∴ good for inpatients as short-term Rx.

- *Promethazine* 25 mg nocte (can ↑dose to 50 mg).

BENZODIAZEPINES

Varying pharmacokinetics are utilised. If shorter-acting, ⇒ ↓hangover/
drowsiness (and ↓accumulation in LF) but ⇒ ↑withdrawal fx when
stopped.

ADVERSE EFFECTS

> ☠*Respiratory depression*☠
> Especially in elderly and if naive to benzodiazepines. Put on close
> nursing observation and monitor O_2 sats if concerned. If using very
> high doses, get iv access and have flumazenil at hand.

- *Dependence/tolerance:* common ∴ prescribe long-term benzodiazepines *only if absolutely necessary* and withdraw ASAP. In order to withdraw safely, if not already on one, swap to long-acting drug (e.g. diazepam) and take 1/8 off the dose every 2 weeks. Try β-blockers to reduce anxiety (avoid antipsychotics).
- *Withdrawal symptoms:* rebound insomnia, tremor, anxiety, confusion, anorexia, toxic psychosis, convulsions, sweating.

Comparison of commonly used benzodiazepines; adapted from www.benzo.org.uk (an excellent resource for information on benzodiazepines), with permission from Professor C.H. Ashton, Institute of Neuroscience, University of Newcastle, UK.

$t_{1/2}$(h)[1]	Drug	Equivalent dose (mg)[1]	Main use(s)
2–3	Midazolam	N/A	Temporary sedation for procedures (titrated iv)
4–15	Oxazepam	20	Good in LF (↓accumulation of metabolites)
6–12	Alprazolam[2]	0.5	Anxiety
6–12	Loprazolam[2]	1–2	Anxiety, insomnia
8–20	Lorazepam	1	Status epilepticus (iv), acute Ψ sedation (im/po)
8–22	Temazepam	20	Insomnia
12–60	Clobazam	20	Epilepsy, anxiety
18–50	Clonazepam	0.5	Movement disorders, epilepsy and Ψ disorders
36–200[3]	Diazepam	10	Status epilepticus (iv/pr), anxiety, alcohol withdrawal
36–200[3]	Chlordiazepoxide	25	Alcohol withdrawal

1 These are approximate and can vary considerably between individuals. 2 Rarely used in the UK.
3 These values are for the active metabolite.

COMBINED HORMONAL CONTRACEPTION

TYPES

- Pills: aka (combined) oral contraceptive pill ((C)OCP):
  - monophasic: fixed quantity of O + P in each tablet;
  - bi/tri phasic: varying quantity of O + P according to cycle stage.
- Patches

Actions

↓s ovulation, Δs cervical mucus (↓s sperm penetration) & Δs
endometrium (⇒ atrophy + ↓s receptiveness to implantation).

Effectiveness

0.2–3 pregnancies/100 woman years (depending on reliability of use).
Indications: Contraception. Also as Rx for some benign gynaeco-
logical conditions, e.g. dysmenorrhoea, menorrhagia & pre-menstrual
syndrome.
CI: FHx of cardiovascular disease, ≤45 yrs old with abnormal lipid or
haemostatic profile, DM (poorly controlled or complications, e.g.
retinopathy), BP ≥160/95 mmHg, smoker (of ≥40/day or ≥35 yrs
old), BMI ≥35, focal or crescendo migraine requiring Rx, Dubin–
Johnson or Rotor syndrome, gallstones, undiagnosed genital tract
bleeding, oestrogen dependent tumours (e.g. breast cancer), medical
conditions that ↑sex steroids (e.g. chorea, pemphigoid gestationis)
L/H/P.
Caution: Heart disease (inc FHx), ≤45 yrs old with normal lipid &
haemostatic profiles, well controlled DM, systolic BP 135–160
mmHg, diastolic BP 85–95 mmHg, smoker (of 5–40 cigarettes/day),
BMI 30–35, uncomplicated migraine, ↑prolactin, severe depression.
SE: Acne, headache, depression, ↑Wt, breast tenderness, thrombus,
↑BP, N&V, abdo cramps, LF, hepatic tumours, fluid retention, Δ lipid
metabolism, chorea, nervousness, irritability, Δ libido, Δ menstrual
pattern, Δ vaginal discharge, cervical erosion, contact lenses irritation,

visual Δ, leg cramps, skin reactions, chloasma, photosensitivity. Rarely gallstones & SLE.

Warn: *Starting*: if starting OCP ≥6 days from 1st day of menses additional contraception should be used for additional 7 days (9 days if low dose oestrogen preparation), or for 14 days after use of ulipristal acetate emergency contraception (16 days if low dose oestrogen preparation). *Missed pills:* If only 1 pill missed it should be taken as soon as remembered and resume normal pill taking; no further action required. If ≥2 pills missed advise to use additional contraception (on top of usual pills) for next 7 days. If these 7 days continue into next packet then pill-free interval should be avoided. *D&V can* ↓↓ *effectiveness*: Additional OCP pill should be taken if V occurs w/in 2 hrs of taking pill. If D&V persists ≥24 hrs additional contraception should be used for next 7 days & next pill free period should be omitted if included in these days. *VTE risk:* ↑risk. (15 in 100 000). NB the absolute risk remains small and significantly < pregnancy risk of VTE (60 in 100 000). Risk ↑with periods of immobility (>5 hrs) associated with travel or recovery for surgery. Appropriate advice prior to long-haul travel would depend on additional risk factors, but should involve exercise and possible use of graduated compression stockings. Prior to major surgery E-containing products should be stopped 4 wks before, and recommenced at the first period, ≥2 wks post-op. Additional contraception should be given during this time.

Interactions: many as **metab by P450**; efficacy ↓ by P450 inducers (see p. 237 and BNF/SPC). Antibiotics can↓ efficacy by Δing bowel flora (e.g. ampicillin, doxycycline).

Choice of preparation

Low strength (Ethinylestradiol 20 microgram) preparations are used if risk factors for **heart failure. Standard strength** (30–35 microgram) preparations are appropriate for most women, however generally best to use preparation with lowest dose giving good cycle control & minimal SEs. Phased preparations may be used if breakthrough bleeding problems with the monophasic pill, or SEs 2° to progestogen effects.

Common combined hormonal contraception preparations

Preparation		Oestrogen (microgram)	Progesterone (mg)	Dose
Low strength oral	Loestin 20	Ethinylestradiol 20	Norethisterone 1	od for 21 days, with 7 days pill free
	Mercilon	Ethinylestradiol 20	Desogestrel 0.15	
	Femodette	Ethinylestradiol 20	Gestodene 0.75	
Standard strength oral	Microgynon 30	Ethinylestradiol 30	Levonorgestrel 0.15	
	Loestrin 30	Ethinylestradiol 30	Norethisterone 1.5	
	Cilest	Ethinylestradiol 35	Norgestimate 0.25	
	Yasmin	Ethinylestradiol 30	Drospirenone 3	
	Femodene	Ethinylestradiol 30	Gestodene 0.075	
Patches	Evra	Ethinylestradiol 33.9/24 h	Norelgestromin 0.203/24 h	1 patch/wk for 3 wks, followed-by 1 patch-free wk

SIDE EFFECT PROFILES

Knowledge of these, together with a drug's mechanism(s), will simplify learning and allow anticipation of drug SEs.

CHOLINOCEPTORS

ACh stimulates nicotinic and muscarinic receptors. Anticholinesterases ⇒ ↑ACh and ∴ stimulate both receptor types and have 'cholinergic fx'. Drugs that ↓cholinoceptor action do so mostly via muscarinic

Cholinergic fx	Antimuscarinic fx
Generally ↑secretions	*Generally* ↓secretions
Diarrhoea	Constipation
Urination	Urinary retention
Miosis (constriction)	Mydriasis ↓accommodation*
Bronchospasm/bradycardia**	Bronchodilation/tachycardia
Excitation of CNS (and muscle)	Drowsiness, **D**ry eyes, **D**ry skin
Lacrimation↑	
Saliva/sweat↑	
Commonly caused by:	
Anticholinesterases:	Atropine, ipratropium (Atrovent)
MG Rx, e.g. pyridostigmine	Antihistamines (inc cyclizine)
Dementia Rx, e.g. rivastigmine, donepezil	Antidepressants (esp TCAs)
	Antipsychotics (esp 'typicals')
	Hyoscine, Ia antiarrhythmics

* ↑blurred vision and ↑IOP. **Together with vasodilation ⇒ ↓BP.

receptors (antinicotinics used only in anaesthesia) and are ∴ more accurately called 'antimuscarinics' rather than 'anticholinergics'.

ADRENOCEPTORS

α generally excites sympathetic system (except*):

- α_1 ⇒ GI smooth-muscle relaxation*, otherwise contracts smooth muscle: vasoconstriction, GI/bladder sphincter constriction (uterus, seminal tract, iris (radial muscle)). Also ↑salivary secretion, ↓glycogenolysis (in liver).
- α_2 ⇒ inhibition of neurotransmitters (esp NA and ACh for feedback control), Pt aggregation, contraction of vascular smooth muscle, inhibition of insulin release. Also prominent adrenoceptor of CNS (inhibits sympathetic outflow).

β generally inhibits sympathetic system (except*):

- β_1 ⇒ ↑HR*, ↑contractility* (and ↑s salivary amylase secretion).

- β_2 ⇒ vasodilation, bronchodilation, muscle tremor, glycogenolysis (in hepatic and skeletal muscle). Also ↑s renin secretion, relaxes ciliary muscle and visceral smooth muscles (GI sphincter, bladder detrusor, uterus if not pregnant).
- β_3 ⇒ lipolysis, thermogenesis (of little pharmacological relevance).

SEROTONIN (5HT)

Relative excess: 'serotonin syndrome'; seen with antidepressants at ↑doses or if swapped without adequate 'tapering' or 'washout period'. Initially causes restlessness, sweating and tremor, progressing to shivering, myoclonus and confusion, and, if severe enough, convulsions/death.

Relative deficit: 'antidepressant withdrawal/discontinuation syndrome' occurs when antidepressants stopped too quickly; likelihood depends on $t_{1/2}$ of drug. Causes 'flu-like' symptoms (chills/sweating, myalgia, headache and nausea), shock-like sensations, dizziness, anxiety, irritability, insomnia, vivid dreams. Rarely ⇒ movement disorders and ↓memory/concentration.

DOPAMINE (DA)

Relative excess: causes behaviour Δ, confusion and psychosis (esp if predisposed, e.g. schizophrenia). Seen with L-dopa and DA agonists used in Parkinson's (and some endocrine disorders, e.g. bromocriptine).

Relative deficit: causes extrapyramidal fx (see below), ↑prolactin (sexual dysfunction, female infertility, gynaecomastia), neuroleptic malignant syndrome. Seen with DA antagonists, esp antipsychotics and certain antiemetics such as metoclopramide, prochlorperazine and levomepromazine.

EXTRAPYRAMIDAL EFFECTS

Abnormalities of movement control arising from dysfunction of basal ganglia.

- *Parkinsonism*: rigidity and bradykinesia ± tremor.
- *Dyskinesias* (= abnormal involuntary movements); commonly:
  - *Dystonia* (= abnormal posture): dynamic (e.g. oculogyric crisis) or static (e.g. torticollis).
  - *Tardive (delayed onset) dyskinesia*: esp orofacial movements.
  - *Others*: tremor, chorea, athetosis, hemiballismus, myoclonus, tics.
- *Akathisia* (= restlessness): esp after large antipsychotic doses.

All are commonly caused by antipsychotics (esp older 'typical' drugs) and are a rare complication of antiemetics (e.g. metoclopramide, prochlorperazine – esp in young women). Dyskinesias and dystonias are common with antiparkinsonian drugs (esp peaks of L-dopa doses).
  Most respond to stopping (or ↓dose of) the drug – if not possible, doesn't work or immediate Rx needed add antimuscarinic drug (e.g. procyclidine) but doesn't work for akathisia (try β-blocker) and can worsen tardive dyskinesia: seek neurology ± psychiatry opinion if in doubt.

CEREBELLAR EFFECTS

Esp antiepileptics (e.g. phenytoin) and alcohol.

- **D**ysdiadokokinesis, dysmetria (= past-pointing) and rebound
- **A**taxia of gait (wide-based, irregular step length) ± trunk
- **N**ystagmus: towards side of lesion; mostly coarse and horizontal
- **I**ntention tremor (also titubation = nodding-head tremor)
- **S**peech: scanning dysarthria – slow, slurred or jerky
- **H**ypotonia (less commonly hyporeflexia or pendular reflexes).

CYTOCHROME P450

Substrates of P450 that often result in significant interactions (these drugs can ↑ severe problems if rendered ineffective or toxic by interactions ∴ always exclude interactions when prescribing!):

- Inhibitors and inducers can affect warfarin, phenytoin, carbamazepine, ciclosporin and theophyllines. Interactions can ∴ ⇒ toxicity **or** treatment failure.
- Inducers affect OCP ∴ can ↑ failure as contraceptive!

> **NB**
> This system is very complex and mediated by many isoenzymes; predicting significant interactions requires understanding which drugs are metabolised by which isoenzymes as well as which, and to what degree, other drugs affect these isoenzymes. Look for **P450** symbols in this book as a rough guide; check SPCs if concerned (available online at www.emc.medicines.org.uk) and for a full overview of the **P450** system see www.edhayes.com/startp450.html.

Medical emergencies

ACUTE CORONARY SYNDROMES (ACS)

Clues: angina, N&V, sweating, LVF (see p. 243), arrhythmias, Hx of IHD. Remember atypical pain and silent infarcts in DM, elderly or if ↓GCS.

ACS encompasses the following:

1   **STEMI:** ST elevation myocardial infarction (see p. 215).
2   **NSTEMI:** Non-ST elevation MI; troponin (T or I) +ve.
3   **UA(P):** Unstable angina (pectoris); troponin (T or I) −ve.

FOR ALL ACS

- Don't routinely administer O_2, but monitor O_2 saturation using pulse oximetry as soon as possible, to guide the use of supplemental oxygen.
- *Aspirin:* 300 mg po stat (chew/dispersible form) unless CI. If in A&E, check has not been given already by paramedics or GP.
- *Clopidogrel:* 300 mg po (some give 600 mg, esp if immediate PCI planned). Prasugrel (60 mg loading dose) and ticagrelor are alternatives – see local guidelines for which to use.
- *Opiate: in UK most centres give diamorphine* 2.5–5 mg iv + antiemetic (e.g. metoclopramide 10 mg iv), repeat diamorphine iv according to response. Morphine is an alternative, initially 3–5 mg iv, repeating every few minutes until pain free.
- *GTN:* 1–2 sprays or sl tablets (max 1.2 mg). If pain continues or LVF develops, set up ivi, titrating to BP and pain. NB: can ⇒ ↓BP; don't give if systolic ≤100 mmHg (esp if combined with ↓BP) or inferior infarct (i.e. suspected RV involvement).

DATE/ TIME	INFUSION FLUID	VOL- UME	ADDITIVES IF ANY DRUG AND DOSE	RATE OF ADMIN	DURA- TION	DR'S SIGNATURE	TIME START- ED	TIME COM- PLETED	SET UP BY SIG- NATURE	BATCH No.
25/12	N. Saline	50 ml	50 mg GTN	0–10 ml/hr*		TN				
	*TITRATE TO PAIN: Stop if systolic BP < 100 mmHg									

Figure 9 Drug chart showing how to write up GTN ivi.

Consider:

- β-blocker: unless CI (see propranolol p. 134), esp beware ☠
  asthma, acute LVF ☠, ↓BP (systolic <100 mmHg), ↓HR
  (<60/min), 2nd-/3rd-degree HB; get senior help if in doubt.
  - *Can be given iv or po:* it is often recommended to give iv for
    STEMI and po for NSTEMI and UAP. In acute settings,
    metoprolol is often drug of choice as short $t_{1/2}$ (if chronic LVF
    use bisoprolol) means it wears off quickly if acute LVF develops.
    Consult local protocol or get senior advice if unsure.
  - *iv:* e.g. metoprolol 1–5 mg iv, giving 1–2 mg aliquots at a time
    while monitoring BP and HR. Repeat to max 15 mg, stopping
    when BP ≤100 mmHg or HR ≤60. Then consider starting
    metoprolol po.
  - *po:* e.g. metoprolol 25–50 mg bd. If cardiodynamically stable
    24 h later, change to long-acting β-blocker, e.g. bisoprolol
    5–10 mg od.
  - If already on β-blocker, ensure dose adequate to control HR.
  - If β-blocker CI and ↑HR consider Ca^{2+} blocker (e.g. diltiazem
    SR 60–120 mg bd) and get senior ± cardiology advice.
- *Insulin:* for all type I DM and type II DM or non-diabetics with
  CBG >11 on admission. Give conventional sliding scale or GIK ivi
  (e.g. DIGAMI) if local protocol exists; contact CCU for advice.
- *iv fluids:* if RV infarct. *Clues:* ↓BP with no pulmonary oedema,
  inferior or posterior ECG Δs (esp ST elevation ≥1 mm in a VF) and
  ↑JVP. If suspected, do right-sided ECG and look for ↑ST in V4.
  Avoid vasodilating drugs (esp nitrates and ACE-i). Care with
  β-blockers (can ⇒ HB).

IF STEMI

- *Reperfusion therapy: primary PCI is the preferred option, if
  unavailable or CI consider thrombolysis.* NB: starting one or
  the other ASAP is paramount ('time = myocardium'!) ∴ if appropriate, initiate/organise during above steps. See p. 215 for thrombolysis indications, CIs and choice of agent.

- *Heparin:* iv heparin is given with *recombinant* thrombolytics for 24–48 h (see p. 215) to avoid the rebound hypercoagulable states they can cause, but is *not* needed with *streptokinase*. If ongoing chest pain or unresolving ECG Δs, get senior advice on further anticoagulation and arrange rescue PCI.
- Consider (consult local protocol/cardiology on-call if unsure):
  - *Glycoprotein IIb/IIIa inhibitor:* esp if not thrombolysed (CI or presentation too late) or PCI planned and still unstable. Use with caution (esp <48 h post-thrombolysis).
  - Rescue PCI: esp if thrombolysis given and doesn't ↓pain (e.g. within 90 min) or non-resolving (e.g ≤50% reduction in) ST elevation on ECG.

IF NSTEMI OR UAP

- *Heparin:* LMWH, e.g. enoxaparin 1 mg/kg bd sc or fondaparinux 2.5 mg od sc esp if PCI planned in 1st 24–36 h after symptom onset.
- Consider (consult local protocol/cardiology on-call if unsure):
  - *Glycoprotein IIb/IIIa inhibitor:* if high risk* (defined by ACC/ESC as: haemodynamic or rhythm instability, persistent pain, acute or dynamic ECG Δs, TIMI risk score >3 (see below), ↓left ventricular function, ↑troponin) and/or ongoing chest pain/ECG Δs.

> TIMI risk score for UA/NSTEMI. (Source: Antman E, et al. JAMA 2000; 284: 835–842).
>
> 1 point for presence of each of the following:
>
> - Age ≥65 yrs
> - ≥3 of following risk factors for IHD: FHx of IHD, ↑BP, ↑cholesterol, DM, current smoker
> - Prior coronary stenosis (≥50% occlusion)
> - Aspirin use in past 7 days
> - Severe angina (≥2 episodes w/in 24 h)
> - ST segment deviations (↑ or ↓) at presentation
> - +ve serum cardiac markers (troponin).

Score >3 indicates ↑risk* of developing cardiac events and death.

SECONDARY PREVENTION

For all ACS unless CI or already started:

- *Next day:* aspirin 75 mg od, 'statin' (e.g. simvastatin 40 mg od) and clopidogrel 75 mg od (for 1 yr[NICE]). If prasugrel used (instead of clopidogrel) 10 mg od unless >75 yrs or <60 kg in which case use 5 mg od.
- *When stable:* β-blocker (if not already started, e.g. bisoprolol 1.25 mg od once any LVF clears; see above for CI) and ACE-i (e.g. ramipril 2.5 mg bd po started 2–10 days after MI, then 5 mg bd after 2 days if tolerated). Consider addition of aldosterone antagonist eplerenone in established LVF (EF <40%) and signs of HF after 3 days (closely monitor U&Es).
- *ASAP:* diet/lifestyle Δs (↓Wt, diet Δs, ↑exercise, ↓smoking, etc).

ACUTE LVF

Clues: SOB, S_3 or S_4, pulmonary oedema (can ⇒ pink frothy sputum if severe), peripheral oedema, ↓BP, Hx of IHD, ↑JVP (if also RVF, i.e. CCF).

- 60–100% O_2 to maintain SaO_2 >95% (care if COPD) and sit patient upright.
- Furosemide 20–40 mg iv initially (max 100 mg in 1st 6 h); consider repeat doses or ivi (5–40 mg/h) later. If not 'in extremis', consider ↓doses (40 or 60 mg) od and monitor urine output.
- Diamorphine 2.5–5 mg iv + metoclopramide 10 mg iv.
- GTN ivi: see ACS section pp. 240.

If patient does not respond/worsens, get senior help and consider:

- *Non-invasive ventilation* (NIV) as continuous positive airways pressure (CPAP). If no machine on ward, find one ASAP!
- *Inotropes:* if ↓BP, e.g. dobutamine (2–20 microgram/kg/min) via central line; if patient is this sick, will also be needed for CVP measurement and CCU care (± intra-aortic balloon pump). Get cardiology advice if needed.

- *?Underlying cause:* MI, arrhythmias (esp AF), ↑↑BP, ↓↓Hb, AKI, anaphylaxis, sepsis, ARDS, poisons/OD (e.g. aspirin).

ACE-i: once stable and if no CI, e.g. enalapril 2.5 mg od (↑later).

ACCELERATED HYPERTENSION

Dx: diastolic >120 mmHg (or systolic >220 mmHg) plus grade III (haemorrhages/exudates) or IV (papilloedema) hypertensive retinopathy. ☠Do not drop BP too quickly as can e.g. ⇒ MI, CVA or AKI☠. NB: patients are often salt and water depleted (look for postural drop of >20 mmHg) so *may require fluid replacement as well as antihypertensives.*

  If life-threatening target organ damage (e.g. encephalopathy, intracranial haemorrhage, aortic dissection, unstable angina, acute MI, acute LVF/pulmonary oedema or pre-eclampsia/eclampsia): get senior help immediately and aim to ↓diastolic to 110–115 mmHg over 1–2 h (systolic to <110 mmHg in aortic dissection) and then more slowly thereafter (e.g. ↓diastolic to 100 mmHg after 48 h). This should always be done in the ITU/HDU/CCU setting and generally (but not always) involve iv antihypertensives; choose from nitroprusside (most commonly used but can ⇒ cyanide poisoning, esp if used in ↓GFR; may not ↓cerebral vascular resistance as well as labetalol), hydralazine (commonly used in pregnancy), labetalol (in pregnancy but can ⇒ severe ↓BP) or phentolamine (esp if phaeo known/suspected). If pulmonary oedema, consider GTN/ISDN.

  If no life-threatening target organ damage (i.e. uncomplicated acute kidney injury, mild LVF, etc): aim to ↓diastolic BP to 110–115 mmHg over 24–48 h using *oral* medication such as:

- Nifedipine (e.g. Adalat Retard) 10 mg po. Monitor and reassess; consider repeat doses (e.g. after 2 h) and if required/tolerated aim to get patient on to higher doses (e.g. 20 mg tds). Tablets to be swallowed (not chewed) and avoid quick release or sl preparations. Convert to amlodipine once stable.
- If IHD consider adding β-blocker* later (e.g. atenolol 25–50 mg od).

- If nifedipine CI, consider diltiazem (e.g. 60 mg SR bd initially) or β-blocker instead*: metoprolol (e.g. 12.5–25 mg initially then tds regimen) or labetalol (e.g. 50–800 mg bd/tds) are good choices as short acting and needs no dose adjustment with ↓GFR. When BP controlled withdraw β-blocker except in IHD (risk of new-onset DM). In IHD consider converting to atenolol (e.g. 50 mg po) once stable.
- Other drugs to consider are ACE-i** (can ⇒ severe ↓BP; if so give iv saline) and diuretics (if patient fluid overloaded).

*If cause is phaeo: will need α-blocker (phenoxybenzamine) and may need salt supplements. If tachycardia a problem, must not give β-blocker until several days after α-blocker started. Suspect if BP very variable, headaches, sweats or palpitations; get senior help.
**Beware: if cause renal artery stenosis (other clinical vascular disease/ multiple CVD risk factors/ ↓GFR) if possible avoid renin system blockade (i.e. ACE-i/ARB/direct renin inhibitor) as ☠ risk of severe ↓BP) and U&Es monitored (risk of RF including delayed onset after 3–4 weeks)☠; if used, starting dose must be low (e.g. enalapril 2.5 mg od).

ATRIAL FIBRILLATION

Clues: ↑HR ± SOB, angina or heart failure. Confirm diagnosis with repeat ECGs; narrow QRS, absent 'P' waves (esp V1), (irregularly) irregular R-R interval.

Treatment (rate and rhythm control) depends on: presence of haemodynamic instability (systolic BP <90 mmHg), acuteness of onset (<48 h) and presence of structural heart disease (e.g. LVH: clinically/ECG/echo) or heart failure (clinically/CXR/echo).

For haemodynamically unstable patients:

- DC cardioversion (see ALS tachycardia algorithm on inside back cover); ideally after initiating anticoagulation* but this shouldn't delay emergency intervention[NICE].

For haemodynamically stable patients:

If acute onset (<48 h)

+ no evidence of structural heart disease: flecainide 100 mg bd po or 2 mg/kg iv over 30 min (max 150 mg) with appropriate antithrombotic cover (e.g. enoxaparin 1.5 mg/kg daily); seek cardiology advice if unsuccessful and consider DC cardioversion.

+ evidence of structural heart disease (or any doubt): amiodarone 300 mg ivi over 20–60 min followed by 900 mg ivi over next 24 h and then 1.2–1.8 g/day (po or iv) until 10 g total. Then minimum maintenance dose (100–400 mg/day) to control sinus rhythm. If unsuccessful consider DC cardioversion.

If onset >48 h (or unknown)

+ no evidence of heart failure: β-blocker po (e.g. metoprolol 25–50 mg bd). If β-blocker CI (e.g. COPD/ asthma) use Ca^{2+} channel blocker (e.g. diltiazem MR 120 mg bd).

+ evidence of heart failure: digoxin 250–500 microgram iv/po loading dose and two repeat half doses at 6–12 h intervals followed by appropriate maintenance dose (62.5–250 microgram). Use half the dose if elderly or RF. Monitor levels and e'lytes to avoid toxicity (see p. 54).

- All inpatients initially need anticoagulation (e.g. LMWH); for paroxysmal, persistent and permanent AF[NICE] use risk stratification for benefit and haemorrhagic risk to guide thromboprophylaxis; high stroke risk[NICE] use warfarin (post stroke/TIA/TE; age ≥75 with HTN, diabetes or vascular disease; structural heart disease or LVF; CHADS$_2$* >3); moderate risk[NICE] use warfarin or aspirin (age ≥65 + no risk factors; age <75 and HTN, diabetes or vascular disease); low risk[NICE] use aspirin.
- If non-acute (planned) cardioversion anticoagulate ≥3 wks before (and after) cardioversion[NICE].

CHADS$_2$ score for risk of stroke in (non-rheumatic) AF: JAMA 2001; : 2864–2870.

- Congestive heart failure Hx = 1 point
- Hypertension Hx   = 1 point

- **Age** ≥ 75 = 1 point
- **DM** Hx = 1 point
- **Stroke** symptoms or TIA = 2 points

ACUTE ASTHMA

Clues: SOB, wheeze, PEF <50% of best**, RR ≥25/min, HR ≥110/min, cannot complete sentences in 1 breath, SaO_2 − ≥92%.
- Attach sats monitor
- 40–60% O_2 through high-flow mask, e.g. Hudson mask
- Salbutamol 5 mg neb in O_2: repeat up to every 15 min if life-threatening
- Ipratropium 0.5 mg neb in O_2: repeat up to every 4 h if life-threatening or fails to respond to salbutamol
- Prednisolone 40–50 mg po od for at least 5 days. Hydrocortisone 100 mg qds iv can be given if unable to swallow or retain tablets.

Both prednisolone and hydrocortisone can be given if very ill.

> *Life-threatening features*
> - PEF <33% of best**
> - O_2 sats <92%
> - PaO_2 <8.0kPa, $PaCO_2$ >4.6kPa or pH <7.35
> - Silent chest, cyanosis or ↓respiratory effort
> - ↓HR, ↓BP or dysrhythmia
> - Exhaustion, confusion or coma
>
> **Or predicted best (see p. 187).

If life-threatening features (NB: patient may not always *appear* distressed), get senior help and consider the following:

- *MgSO₄ ivi:* 1.2–2 g over 20 min (8 mmol = 2 g = 4 ml of 50% solution) unlicensed indication.
- *Aminophylline iv:* attach cardiac monitor and give loading dose* of 5 mg/kg iv over 20 min then ivi at 0.5–0.7 mg/kg/h (0.3 mg/kg/h if

elderly). ☠ **If already on maintenance po aminophylline/
theophylline, omit loading dose* and check levels ASAP to guide
dosing** ☠ .

- *ivi salbutamol:* 5 microgram/min initially (then up to
  20 microgram/min according to response): back-to-back or
  continuous nebs now often preferred.
- Call anaesthetist for consideration of ITU care or intubation.
  Initiate this during the above steps if deteriorating.

COPD EXACERBATION

Clues: SOB, wheeze, RR >25/min, HR >110.

- *Attach sats monitor* and do baseline ABGs.
- *28% O_2 via Venturi mask;* should be *prescribed on drug chart.*
  ↑dose cautiously if hypoxia continues, but repeat ABGs to ensure
  CO_2 not ↑ing and (more importantly) pH not ↓ing.
- *Ipratropium 0.5 mg neb* in O_2: repeat up to every 4 h if very ill.
- *Salbutamol 5 mg neb* in O_2: repeat up to every 15 min if very ill
  (seldom necessary >hourly).
- *Prednisolone 30 mg po* then od for ≤2 wks (often 7–10 days).
  Some give 1st dose as hydrocortisone 200 mg iv – rarely used now
  unless unable to swallow.
- *Antibiotics* (see p. 175) if 2 out of 3 of Hx of ↑ing SOB, ↑ing
  volume or ↑ing purulence of sputum.

If no improvement, consider:

- *Aminophylline ivi:* see Mx of asthma (p. 247) for details.
- Assisted ventilation: CPAP if just ↓PaO_2 or NIV (BIPAP) if also
  ↑PaCO_2; consider doxapram if NIV not available.
- Intubation: discuss with ITU/anaesthetist.

PULMONARY EMBOLISM

Clues: unlikely unless RR >20 and PaO_2 <10.7kPa (or ↓O_2 sats).

- *60–100% O_2* if hypoxic. Care if COPD.

- *Analgesia:* if xs pain or distress, try paracetamol/ibuprofen 1st; consider opiates if severe or no response (☠ can ⇒ respiratory depression☠).
- *Anticoagulation:* LMWH, e.g. dalteparin or enoxaparin. Once PE confirmed, load with warfarin (see pp. 207). Consider iv heparin if surgery being contemplated, or rapid reversal may be required*.

If massive PE, worsening hypoxia or cardiovascular instability (↓BP, RV strain/failure), seek senior help and consider:

- *Fluids ± inotropes:* if systolic BP <90 mmHg
- *Thrombolysis (e.g. alteplase):* if ↓BP ± collapse
- *Embolectomy*:* seek urgent cardiothoracic opinion.

ACUTE UPPER GI HAEMORRHAGE

Clues: Haematemesis and/or melaena; consider as differential in sudden collapse/shock.

Assess severity of bleeding

- Pulse >100 or ↑ of >20bpm
- Systolic BP <100 mmHg (or postural drop >10 mmHg)
- Cold, clammy peripheries
- Urine output <0.5 ml/kg/h (30ml/h).

Management

- Resuscitate:
  - Give high-flow O_2
  - Insert 2 wide bore intravenous cannulae (grey/brown)
  - iv fluid (blood *or* colloid *or* crystalloid) to maintain systolic BP >100
  - Correct clotting with iv fresh frozen plasma if INR >1.5
    (**NB:** Vit K reverses warfarin but doesn't affect clotting problems due to synthetic liver function abnormalities).
- Take blood for:
  - FBC, INR, U&E, LFT
  - Group and save or cross match 2–6 units depending on severity of bleed.

- Monitor (at least hourly):
  - Pulse, BP, urine output (consider catheter)
  - Consider CVP for elderly or suspected variceal bleed.
- Drugs:
  - **Stop** antihypertensives, diuretics, NSAIDs, anticoagulants
  - In severe non-variceal bleed, give omeprazole 40 mg iv
  - Give 2 mg terlipressin iv 'stat' if variceal bleed suspected (and continue qds – NB: caution in IHD)
  - All suspected variceal bleeds should receive a short course of prophylactic antibiotics active against Gram negative bacteria.
- Endoscopy: indicated urgently if:
  - Variceal bleed suspected

Rockall score (*Gut* 1996; **38**: 316–321).

		Score			
	Variable	0	1	2	3
Pre-OGD Score	Age	<60	60–79	>80	
	Shock	sBP >100; HR <100	sBP >100; HR <100	sBP <100;	
	Comorbidity	nil major		HF, IHD, or any major comorbidity	RF, LF, disseminated malignancy
Post-OGD Score	Diagnosis	Mallory-Weisstear, no lesion, no SRH	All other Dx	Malignancy of upper GI tract	
	Major SRH	None or dark spot only		Blood in upper GI tract, adherent clot, visible or spurting vessel	

OGD=Oesophago gastro duodenoscopy; sBP = systolic blood pressure; SRH = stigmata of recent haemorrhage.

Pre-OGD score 0 or 1 assoc with <2.5% mortality; can usually be safely endoscoped on the next available list (but w/in 24 hours).

Pre-OGD score >2 assoc with >5% mortality; may require urgent endoscopy.

- Continued bleeding requiring >4 units blood to maintain systolic BP >100 mmHg
- Re-bleed after resuscitation
- Consider if 'Rockall' pre-OGD score ≥2 (see *below*).

SEPSIS (SEVERE OR SEPTIC SHOCK)

Clues: evidence of infection + ↓BP (MAP <65 mmHg), serum lactate >4 mmol/l or ↓urine output

- Oxygen: 100% via non-rebreathe mask (caution if COPD).
- Fluid: 1 litre of crystalloid (or 300–500ml of colloid bolus) over 30 min; if still ↓BP measure CVP and consider further iv fluids (20 ml/kg) to achieve CVP ≥8 mmHg and urine output >0.5 ml/kg/h (caution if LVF).
- Inotropes: if systolic BP <90 mmHg after fluid resuscitation start noradrenaline (1–10 microgram/min) to maintain MAP >65 mmHg. Measure mixed venous O_2 saturation and if <65–70% need further fluid/packed RBCs to achieve haematocrit >30%.
- Antibiotics: as appropriate (see pp. 172) ASAP (w/in 1 h) ensuring all cultures taken 1st (unless significantly delays antibiotics).
- Steroids: consider iv hydrocortisone (200–300 mg/day) when ↓BP responds poorly to adequate fluid resuscitation and vasopressors.
- Activated protein C: consider if multiorgan dysfunction, ↑risk of death (e.g. Acute Physiology and Chronic Health Evaluation (APACHE) II score >25) and no CIs.
- Blood products: aim for Hb >10 g/dl to maximise tissue perfusion.
- Blood glucose: aim for <8.3 mmol/l using validated insulin sliding scale.
- Deep vein thrombosis prophylaxis: low-dose LMWH (e.g enoxaparin 40 mg sc od) unless CI.
- Stress ulcer prophylaxis: H_2 antagonist or PPI.

Adapted from Surviving Sepsis Campaign: International guidelines for management of severe sepsis and septic shock: 2008. *Intensive Care Medicine* 2008; **34**(1).

EPILEPSY

Status epilepticus = seizure lasting >30 min **or** multiple seizures lasting >30 min without full recovery between episodes. NB: 5 min has been suggested as more suitable definition than 30 min. Mortality: 35% if seizures last > 1 hr; 4% if last < 30 min.

> *NB*
> Non-convulsive/absence seizures are missed easily. Keep in mind non-epileptic (='pseudo') seizures, esp if atypical fits.

- Protect airway with tracheal intubation if necessary: call anaesthetist early if concerned.
- Attach O_2 sats, ECG and BP monitors and place in recovery position.
- Give high-flow O_2 via Hudson mask.
- Exclude or treat reversible metabolic causes: esp ↓O_2, ↓glucose (remember to give thiamine if treating ↓glucose in alcoholic or malnourished patient).
- Lorazepam 4 mg iv over 2 min (terminates 60–90% of status epilepticus). If not available use diazepam 10 mg iv over 2 min. If no iv access consider midazolam 5–10 mg im.
- Check BP: maintain or ↑mean arterial BP to provide appropriate cerebral perfusion pressure.

If seizures continue get senior help.

- Repeat lorazepam 4 mg iv over 2 min (or alternative as above).

If no response after 5 min, call for anaesthetist, and give:

- Phenytoin initially total dose 18 mg/kg ivi with normal saline (not compatible with glucose) at 25–50 mg/min then adjust (see p. 129. Fosphenytoin iv is an alternative: see p. 74 for dose as different to phenytoin). Monitor BP and HR (both can drop) and ECG (esp QTc, as arrhythmias not uncommon). Phenytoin will abort 60% of status epilepticus not terminated by lorazepam.

If seizures persist, phenobarbital (15 mg/kg ivi) at 100 mg/min should be considered. If already taking phenytoin po (and plasma levels assumed adequate) consider giving phenobarbital before phenytoin ivi; get senior advice if required.

If the above measures do not terminate seizures, refractory status epilepticus is present. Requires general anaesthesia with propofol and/or thiopental in a specialised unit, often with EEG monitoring.

DKA

Clues: ketotic breath, Kussmaul's (deep/rapid) breathing, dehydration, confusion/↓GCS.

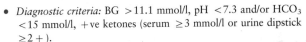

'The Joint British Diabetes Societies Inpatient Care Group has recently published UK guidelines for the Mx of DKA in adults (http://eng.mapofmedicine.com/evidence/map/diabetes4.html). These involve using a fixed rate insulin ivi rather than sliding scale, use of blood ketone measurement to guide treatment, use of bedside glucose and ketone meters when available, and use of venous rather than arterial blood gases. This guidance is increasingly being incorporated into local guidelines, and this section has been updated to reflect it. *NB: follow local diabetes team protocols where applicable; the below guidance is an example of a guideline for DKA Mx'.*

- *Diagnostic criteria:* BG >11.1 mmol/l, pH <7.3 and/or HCO_3 <15 mmol/l, +ve ketones (serum ≥3 mmol/l or urine dipstick ≥2+).
- *Initial measures:* O_2 if hypoxic, weigh patient (if possible), 2 wide bore iv cannulae. Consider NGT (if coma) and central line (esp if ↓↓pH or Hx of HF), but urinary catheter often sufficient.
- *Initial Ix:* blood ketones, CBG, venous BG, U&Es, venous blood gases (ABG if hypoxic), FBC, CRP, blood cultures, ECG, CXR, urinalysis and culture.
- *Biochemical monitoring:* hourly CBG and ketones (bedside if available), venous blood gas (for pH, bicarbonate and K^+) hourly for 1st 2 h, then 2-hourly.

- *Iv fluids:* initially 0.9% saline according to individual patient needs (guided by pulse, BP, urine output $\pm$ CVP). The following is a guide:
  - *If systolic BP <90 mmHg:* 500 ml over 15 min. If BP remains <90 mmHg repeat this but call for senior help.
  - *Otherwise* give more slowly, e.g. 1 litre over 1 h, then 2 litres over 4 h, then 2 litres over 8 h.
  - Add KCl once K^+ <5.5 mmol/l, as can $\downarrow$ rapidly dt insulin (but do not give KCl in 1st litre unless K^+ <3.5 mmol/l). Roughly 40 mmol needed per litre during rehydration: adjust to individual response with regular checks (quickest done with blood gas machines: most give K^+ levels; can use venous samples as long as put in ABG or other heparinised syringe).
- *Insulin:* as soluble insulin ivi (e.g. Actrapid). Use a fixed rate ivi 0.1 units/kg/h (estimate Wt if necessary). Fx: $\downarrow$BG (aim $\downarrow$BG by 3 mmol/l/h), $\downarrow$ketogenesis (aim $\downarrow$blood ketones 0.5 mmol/l/h; if no ketone measurement: aim $\uparrow$bicarbonate 3 mmol/l/h), $\downarrow K^+$ (keep between 4 and 5 mmol/l). If delay in ivi availability, give 0.1 units/kg im stat ($\downarrow$dose if BG <20 mmol/l). If patient takes long-acting insulin sc (Lantus or Levemir) continue this at usual dose/time. If blood ketones not $\downarrow$ing to target, $\uparrow$insulin ivi rate by 1 unit/h. Once BG <14 add 10% glucose 125 ml/h alongside 0.9% saline. If BG <7 do not stop insulin but $\uparrow$rate of glucose ivi. Continue insulin ivi until blood ketones cleared, pH normal and eating/drinking; then switch to sc regimen (see p. 205 for advice).
- *Heparin:* give LMWH until mobile; follow local guidelines.

Consider:

- *Antibiotics:* search for and treat infection.
- *Diabetes specialist team:* involve ASAP.
- *Pregnancy test:* for presentation of gestational diabetes.
- *HDU/ITU:* for one-to-one nursing $\pm$ ventilation if required.
- *Bicarbonate:* if severe acidosis (e.g. pH <7); very rarely needed and potentially dangerous. Get senior help if concerned.

Watch for complications: *e'lyte* Δs (esp ↓K^+, ↓Na^+, ↓Mg^{2+}, ↓PO_4), TE (esp DVT/PE), *cerebral oedema* (↓GCS, papilloedema, false-localising cranial nerve palsies), ARDS, *infections* (esp aspiration pneumonia).

HONK

Clues: as for DKA, but no ketones, normal pH, ↑glucose, ↑dehydration and ↑confusion. Key features are severe hyperglycaemia and hyperosmolality (usually >340 mOsmol/l; calculate using $2(K^+ + Na^+)$ + urea + BG, all in mmol/l). Generally ↑age of patient and ↑length of Hx of decline/insidious onset (NB: may be 1st presentation and no past Hx). May be precipitated by intercurrent illness or drugs (e.g. steroids, thiazides).

- *Initial measures:* as DKA; see above.
- *iv fluids:* as DKA, but can correct dehydration more slowly (will have occurred more slowly and also ↓s risk of e'lyte abnormalities). A rough guide is 1 litre of 0.9% saline over 1 h, then 2 litres over 4 h × 2, then 1 litre over 4 h. Less KCl will be needed, as less insulin will be used. NB: can remain in circulatory collapse despite clinically adequate fluid replacement; if so, give 500ml colloid and monitor CVP. Consider 0.45% saline if Na^+ >155 mmol/l but get senior (ideally specialist) help first as rapid ↓osmolality can ⇒ cerebral oedema.
- *Insulin:* commence insulin ivi; start at lower dose than DKA, e.g. 2 or 3 units/h. Aim to ↓BG by 3–6 mmol/l/h and continue ivi for >24 h (adding glucose if necessary to keep BG normal). Seek early senior help and follow local protocols. Sliding scale insulin may be required. Discuss with diabetes team, including need for subsequent sc insulin.
- *Heparin:* usually LMWH (see pp. 212). Always give, as ↑↑osmolality ⇒ ↑risk of TE (and consider TEDS).

Consider:

- *Antibiotics:* search for and treat infection, as above.
- Watch for complications, esp TE (CVA, IHD), AKI, cerebral oedema.

↓GLUCOSE

Treat if <3 mmol/l or symptoms: ↑sympathetic drive (↑HR, sweating, aggression/behavioural Δs), seizures or confusion/↓GCS.

- *Glucose orally:* esp sugary drinks, mouth gel (e.g. hypostop/ glucogel) or dextrose tablets. Miss this step if severe, but useful if delays in iv access.
- *Glucose 20–50 ml of 50% iv stat* via large iv cannula. Always flush liberally with saline as 50% glucose is very viscous and will act slowly otherwise. Repeat if necessary. A brisk 5–20% glucose ivi can be used if only mild symptoms or until 50% glucose found; beware of fluid overload if HF.
- *Glucagon 1 mg im/iv stat:* if very low glucose or no iv access. Give oral carbohydrate within 10–30 min to prevent recurrence.

NB: think of and correct any causes, esp xs DM Rx, alcohol withdrawal, liver failure, aspirin OD (rarely Addison's disease, ↓T₄). If dt sulphonylureas, relapse is common; consider admission.

THYROTOXIC CRISIS

Clues: ↑HR/AF, fever, abdominal pain, D&V, tremor, agitation, confusion, coma. Look for goitre, Graves' eye disease, Hx of ↓compliance with antithyroid Rx. May be precipitated in a thyrotoxic patient by intercurrent illness/trauma/surgery.

- *O_2:* if hypoxic.
- *0.9% saline ivi:* slowly as per individual needs (care if HF).
- *Propranolol 40 mg tds po:* aim for HR <100 and titrate up dose if necessary (if β-blocker CI, give diltiazem 60–120 mg qds po). If ↑↑HR, give propranolol iv 1 mg over 1 min, repeating if necessary every 2 min to max total of 10 mg.
- *Carbimazole:* 15–30 mg qds po (↓later under specialist advice).
- *Lugol's solution (iodine):* 0.1–0.3 ml tds po (normally for 1 wk). Start 4 h after carbimazole. Blocks T_4 release from gland.
- *Hydrocortisone:* 100 mg qds iv (or dexamethasone 4 mg qds po). ↓s T_4 ⇒ T_3 conversion.

Consider:

- *Treat any heart failure* (common if fast AF), e.g. furosemide.
- *Digoxin and LMWH* (if AF): DC shock rarely works until euthyroid.
- *Antibiotics:* if evidence/suspicion of infection.
- *Cooling measures:* paracetamol, sponging.

If vomiting, insert NGT to avoid aspiration and for drug administration.

MYXOEDEMA COMA

Clues: 'facies', goitre, thyroidectomy scar, ↓temperature, ↓HR, ↓reflexes, ↓glucose, seizures, coma. NB: Ψ features common.

- *O₂:* if hypoxic; protect airway.
- *Monitor pulse, BP:* watch for ↓HR, ↓BP, HF.
- *Glucose iv:* if hypoglycaemic (often coexists); see p. 256.
- *0.9% saline ivi:* slowly as per individual needs (care if HF).
- *Liothyronine* (= T₃ = tri-iodothyronine): 5–20 microgram ivi bd for >2 days then ↑dose with endocrinologist's advice before converting to thyroxine po. Liothyronine can precipitate angina; ↓ rate ivi if occurs. Thyroxine is sometimes given 1st line instead.
- *Hydrocortisone:* 100 mg iv tds, until hypopituitarism excluded (↑likely if no goitre or past Hx of Rx for ↑T₄).

Consider:

- *Rewarming measures:* e.g. Bair-Hugger, warm iv fluids (and O₂).
- *Antibiotics:* infections are common and may have precipitated decline ∴ have low threshold for aggressive Rx.
- *Ventilation/ITU:* condition has high mortality.

ADDISONIAN CRISIS

Clues: ↓BP, ↑HR, ↓glucose, ↑K⁺/↓Na⁺, Hx of chronic high-dose steroid Rx with missed doses or intercurrent illness*.

- O_2 if hypoxic.
- *Glucose iv*: if hypoxic; see p. 256.
- *Steroids*: usually hydrocortisone 100 mg iv stat then qds (ensure blood sample for cortisol and ACTH taken before first dose if Dx is not certain). Give 1st dose as dexamethasone 8 mg iv if Synacthen test planned (hydrocortisone affects test results). Consider fludro-cortisone once stable.
- *Fluids iv*: 0.9% saline $\pm$ central line if $\downarrow\downarrow$BP.
- *Antibiotics*: look for and treat infection*: dipstick urine, MSU, CXR and blood cultures. If in doubt, start Rx.

NB: Check other pituitary hormones in case of associated other pituitary dysfunction.

ELECTROLYTE DISTURBANCES

↑K$^+$

K^+ >6 mmol/l considered dangerous. *Is haemolysis of sample possible cause?* Ring lab $\pm$ repeat sample if suspicious.

If K^+ >6.5 mmol/l or ECG Δs (tall tented T waves, QRS >0.12 sec (>3 small squares), loss of P waves or sinusoidal pattern) the following is needed:

- *Attach cardiac monitor* (+ECG if possible): risk of arrhythmias.
- *10ml of 10% Ca^{2+} gluconate* iv over 3 min for 'cardioprotection', or 10 ml of 10% CaCl iv at $\leq$1ml/min (often found in crash trolleys).
- *10 units insulin* (e.g. Actrapid) + 50 ml 50% glucose ivi over 30 min: stimulates cellular membrane H$^+$/K$^+$ pumps $\therefore$ $\downarrow$s plasma K^+ levels. Beware of too rapid a drop as this may precipitate arrhythmias: aim for drop of 1–2 mmol/l over 30–60 min.
- Consider *salbutamol 5–20 mg nebs*: utilises K$^+$-lowering fx.

For all patients with $\uparrow K^+$:

- *Look for and treat causes*, esp AKI (consider dialysis) and drugs; e.g. iv KCl, oral K^+ supplements, ACE-i, ARBs, K^+-sparing diuretics, NSAIDs. Also ciclosporin but don't adjust without specialist advice.

If $\uparrow K^+$ persists:

- Assess fluid balance and whether passing urine (uric); if not uric total body K^+ won't $\downarrow$ with the above measures and plasma K^+ will eventually return to former levels.
- Consider kaliuretic agents (diuretics not K^+-sparing) if uric.

NB: Contrary to dogma Calcium Resonium is not useful.

$\downarrow K^+$

<2.5 mmol/l $\Rightarrow$ risk of arrhythmias: attach cardiac monitor.

- *1 litre normal saline (0.9%) + 40 mmol KCl* over 4 h. If unstable or arrhythmias develop, seek senior help. KCl can be given quicker but non-specialist wards may not allow >10 mmol/h and patient may not tolerate fast peripheral ivi due to pain (consider central line).
- *Oral K^+ replacement* should also be commenced (e.g. Sando-K, Slow-K 2 tablets tds, or as much as can be tolerated – unpleasant taste!). Beware of overshooting later, esp if cause removed.

NB: po replacement is often sufficient if K^+ >2.5 mmol/l and no clinical features/ECG Δs (small T waves or large U waves).

$\uparrow Ca^{2+}$

>2.65 mmol/l is abnormal. Symptoms usually start once >2.9 mmol/l. *Clues:* bones (pain, esp consider metastases), stones (renal colic $\pm$ AKI), groans (abdominal pains, constipation $\pm$ vomiting; polyuria and thirst common) and psychic moans (inc confusion).

If >3.5 mmol/l or severe symptoms treat urgently as follows:

- 0.9% *saline ivi*: average requirements 4–6 litres over 24 h ($\downarrow$ if elderly/HF). Monitor fluid balance carefully and correct electrolytes.

If insufficient improvement in Ca^{2+} levels or symptoms get senior help and consider:

- *Loop diuretic* (e.g. furosemide): consider once rehydrated.
- *Bisphosphonate* (e.g. pamidronate) esp if $\uparrow$PTH or malignancy.
- *Calcitonin*: if no response to bisphosphonate.
- *Steroids*: if sarcoid, lymphoma, myeloma or vitamin D toxicity.
- *Dialysis*: if AKI or life-threatening symptoms.

OVERDOSES

Unless you are familiar with the up-to-date Mx of the specific overdose in question, the following sources should always be consulted:

- *Toxbase website (www.toxbase.org)*: authoritative and updated regularly. Should be used in the 1st instance to check clinical features and Mx of the poison(s) in question. You will need to sign in under your departmental account; if your department is not registered, contact your A&E department to obtain a username and password.
- *National Poisons Information Service (NPIS)*: if in UK phone 0844 892 0111 (if in Ireland 01 809 2566) for advice if unsure of Toxbase instructions and for rarer/mixed overdoses.

GENERAL MEASURES

- *Activated charcoal*: if w/in 1 h of significant ingestion. CI if $\downarrow$GCS (unless ET tube *in situ*), or if bowel sounds absent or if corrosive substance/petroleum ingested. Repeated doses and administration later than 1 h considered for certain drugs (e.g. quinine, carbamazepine, theophylline, or sustained release preparations). Charcoal not effective for lithium, iron, organophosphates, ethylene glycol, ethanol, methanol.

- *Gastric lavage:* Rarely used, but may be used if w/in 1 h of life-threatening ingestion. CI ↓GCS (unless airway protected), or if corrosive ingested or risk of GI haemorrhage/perforation.
- See Toxbase for dosage guide for activated charcoal, and consult Toxbase ± NPIS for severe or unusual poisoning, as routine GI decontamination is no longer recommended.
- Check paracetamol and aspirin levels in all patients who are unable to give an accurate Hx of the exact poisons ingested.

PARACETAMOL

Significant OD = ingestion of 150 mg/kg or 12 g (whichever is smaller) within 24 h. If risk factors (see below), 75 mg/kg should be used instead.

> *Risk factors in paracetamol OD*
>
> - Taking enzyme-inducing drugs, e.g. carbamazepine, phenobarbital, primidone, phenytoin, rifampicin, St John's wort.
> - Regularly consumes alcohol in xs of recommended amounts.
> - Malnourished and likely to be glutathione-deplete, e.g. anorexia, alcoholism, cystic fibrosis, HIV infection, acute starvation.

Initial management

This depends on time since ingestion. 0–8 h post-ingestion:

- *Activated charcoal:* if w/in 1 h of significant OD.
- *Acetylcysteine:* wait until 4 h post-ingestion before taking urgent sample for paracetamol levels (results are meaningless until this time). If presents at 4–8 h post-ingestion, take sample ASAP.

If levels above the treatment line (see below), give the following
acetylcysteine regimen:
- *Initially* 150 mg/kg in 200 ml 5% glucose ivi over 15 min.
- *Then* 50 mg/kg in 500 ml 5% glucose ivi over 4 h.
- *Then* 100 mg/kg in 1000 ml 5% glucose ivi over 16 h.

NB: if patient weighs >110 kg, use 110 kg (rather than their actual
weight) for these calculations.

> Do not delay acetylcysteine beyond 8 h post-ingestion if waiting for
> paracetamol level and significant OD (beyond 8 h, efficacy ↓s
> substantially) – ivi can be stopped if levels come back as below
> treatment line and INR, ALT and creatinine normal.

8–15 h post-ingestion:

- *Acetylcysteine:* give above regimen ASAP if significant OD taken.
  Do not wait for urgent paracetamol level result. Acetylcysteine can
  be stopped if level later turns out to be below treatment line and
  timing of the OD is certain and patient asymptomatic with normal
  INR, creatinine and ALT.

15–24 h post-ingestion:

- *Acetylcysteine:* give above regimen ASAP unless certain that
  significant OD has not been taken. Do not wait for paracetamol
  level result. Presenting this late ⇒ severe risk, and treatment lines
  are unreliable: always finish course of acetylcysteine.

>24 h post-ingestion:

- Acetylcysteine is controversial when presenting this late. Check
  creatinine, LFTs, INR, glucose, and paracetamol concentration,
  and consult Toxbase or NPIS re individual cases.

NB: use high-risk line if any of the risk factors above apply.

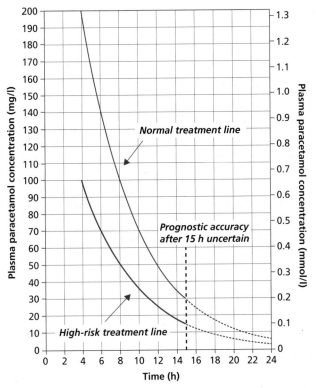

Figure 10 Treatment lines for acetylcysteine treatment of paracetamol overdose. Reproduced courtesy of Alun Hutchings and University of Wales College of Medicine Therapeutics and Toxicology Centre.

> *Important points regarding acetylcysteine*
>
> - Have lower threshold for initiating Rx if doubts over timing of OD, if ingestion was staggered, if presents 24–36 h post-ingestion, or if evidence of LF/severe toxicity regardless of time since ingestion. Contact NPIS if unsure.
> - Anaphylactoid reactions common esp at initial faster rates. Reduce infusion rate or stop temporarily until reaction settles. Give antihistamine (e.g. chlorphenamine 10–20 mg iv over 1 min) if required. Give salbutamol nebs if significant bronchospasm. Once reaction settles restart acetylcysteine, and consider giving the second bag at half normal rate (i.e. 50 mg/kg over 8 h). Past Hx of such reactions is not an absolute CI to future treatment. Pretreatment with chlorphenamine 10 mg iv **or** administration of 1st ivi at slower rate (e.g. over 1 h rather than 15 min) may reduce risk of reaction but the latter is **unlicensed**.
> - Acetylcysteine ⇒ mildly ↑INR itself; ∴ if after treatment ALT is normal but INR is ≤1.3 no further monitoring or treatment is needed. But if ALT is ↑continue acetylcysteine ivi at rate of 150 mg/kg given over 24 h (unless substantial pause in ivi further loading dose not needed).

Subsequent management

Patients may be *medically* fit for discharge once acetylcysteine ivi is completed, and INR, ALT, creatinine and HCO_3^- ($\pm$pH) are normal (or recovering in two successive checks if additional acetylcysteine has been administered). *Psychiatric* evaluation should be undertaken for all patients who have taken a deliberate overdose.

In patients with laboratory abnormalities despite acetylcysteine, consult Toxbase $\pm$ NPIS for advice on further acetylcysteine and specialist referral.

ASPIRIN

- *Consider activated charcoal $\pm$ gastric lavage:* if w/in 1 h of OD of >125 mg/kg. Aspirin delays gastric emptying (esp if enteric-coated tablets), ∴ both can be considered >1 h after ingestion and activated charcoal can be repeated every 4 hrs if salicylate levels continue to rise despite measures below; consult Toxbase for activated charcoal dose and contraindications.

- *Monitor* U&Es, glucose, clotting, ABGs (or venous pH and HCO_3^-) and fluid balance (often need large volumes of iv fluid). Salicylate levels needed if OD of >120 mg/kg; take sample at least 2 h post-ingestion if symptomatic or 4 h post-ingestion if not symptomatic, repeating in both cases 2 h later if severe toxicity suspected in case of delayed absorption (repeating until levels ↓). Note that peak concentrations are often delayed after large ingestions.

If significant biochemical abnormalities, get senior help or contact ITU for specialist advice, and then consider the following:

- *Sodium bicarbonate:* Consider 1.5 litres of 1.26% iv over 2 h (or 225 ml of 8.4%) if metabolic acidosis and salicylate levels >500 mg/l (3.6 mmol/l). This will minimise movement of salicylate into tissues, and enhance renal elimination. Ensure given through patent cannula (risk of tissue necrosis if extravasation). Bicarbonate administration may cause hypokalaemia: monitor K^+ closely. Monitor arterial blood gases to ensure correction of acid–base disturbance, and re-check serum salicylate concentrations.
- *Haemodialysis:* if salicylate levels >700 mg/l (5.1 mmol/l) or unresponsive to the above measures. Also consider if AKI, CCF, non-cardiac pulmonary oedema, severe metabolic acidosis, convulsions or any CNS fx that are not resolved by correction of pH, and in patients aged >70 yrs due to increased risk of toxicity.

OPIATES

Clues: pinpoint pupils, ↓respiratory rate, ↓GCS, drug chart and Hx/signs of opiate abuse (e.g. collapsed vein 'track marks').

- O_2+maintain airway ± ventilatory support.
- *Naloxone 0.4–2 mg iv* (or im) stat initially, repeating after 2 min if no response (check pupils). See p. 114 for subsequent dosing. Note that large doses (>2 mg) may be required in some patients.

BENZODIAZEPINES

- O_2 + maintain airway $\pm$ ventilatory support.
- Consider *flumazenil only if access to ventilatory support is likely to be delayed:* see pp. 54 for dosage.

> 💀 Flumazenil is not recommended as a diagnostic test and should not be given routinely 💀. Risk of inducing fits (esp if epileptic or habituated to benzodiazepines) and arrhythmia (esp if co-ingested TCA or amphetamine-like drug of abuse). If in any doubt, get senior help.

Reference information

COMA

Glasgow Coma Scale (GCS): standardised assessment of coma.

Motor response	Verbal response	Eye opening
6 Obeys commands	5 Orientated	4 Spontaneous
5 Localises pain	4 Confused	3 Responds to speech
4 Withdraws to pain	3 Inappropriate	2 Responds to pain
3 Flexes to pain	2 Incomprehensible	1 None
2 Extends to pain	1 None	
1 No response to pain		

- GCS 13–15 = minor injury
- GCS 9–12 = moderate injury
- GCS <9   = severe injury

NB: drops of >2 are often significant.

To remember GCS use **MoVE** for 3 categories and mnemonic
'OLDFEZ OCEAN SOON', visualising an old fez (Moroccan hat)
floating down a river that will soon arrive at the ocean!

- **Motor:** Obeys, Localises, Draws away, Flexor, Extensor, Zero.
- **Verbal:** Orientated, Confused, Explicit (or e**X** rated), Absolute
  rubbish, None.
- **Eye:** Spontaneous, Orders only, Ouch only, None.

> **Causes of ↓GCS = DIM TOPS**
> - *Drugs:* alcohol, insulin, sedatives, overdoses (esp opiates/benzo-
>   diazepines).
> - *Infections:* sepsis, meningitis, encephalitis.
> - *Metabolic:* ↑/↓glucose, ↓T_4, Addison's, renal/liver failure.
> - *Trauma Hx:* unwitnessed fall or extradural 'lucid interval'.
> - *O_2 deficiency:* any cause of ↓O_2 (NB: ↑CO_2 is also a cause).
> - *Perfusion:* CVA (inc SAH), MI, PE/Pressure: ↑ICP.
> - *Seizures:* post-ictal fx and non-convulsive status aren't obvious.

COGNITIVE IMPAIRMENT

1 **(A)MTS:** (Abbreviated) Mental Test Score – most basic assessment of cognition; popular with physicians due to brevity (esp for use on the elderly). <8/10 is abnormal (i.e. dementia and/or delirium).

W   World War II: what year did it end?[1]
H   Hospital (what is name of building you are in?).
A   Address: 42 West St (ask to repeat and remember*).
T   Time: to the nearest hour.
Y   Year.
E   Elizabeth II (who is current monarch?)[1].
A   Age (of patient).
R   Recognition of 2 persons: e.g. Dr and other[2].
B   Birthday (patient's date of birth).
C   Count backwards from 20 to 1.
?   ? Can you remember the address?*.

[1]If culturally inappropriate change to relevant question or omit.
[2]If alone with patient omit.

If questions omitted, record why and reduce denominator of score.

2 **MMSE:** Mini Mental State Examination; popular and best validated basic cognitive assessment. **Questions to ask are in bold.**

Orientation:
Time – (1–3) **Date?** 1 point for each for day, month and year.   5
(4) **Season?** (5) **Day of week?**
Place – (1) **Country?** (2) **County/state (or large city)?**   5
(3) **Town (or city area)?** (4) **Building?** (5) **Floor?**
Registration: Say[1] **ball, flag, tree.** Repeat until success or   3
5 attempts.
Attention/concentration: **Spell 'WORLD' backwards**[2].   5
Recall: **Can you remember those 3 items?** (ball, flag, tree).   3
3-stage command: **Take paper in R hand, fold in half and put**   3
on floor.
Language: **What is this?** Point to pen and then wristwatch.   2

Repeat exactly after me: 'No ifs, ands or buts.'   1
Reading/comprehension: Do what the sentence below instructs[3].   1
Praxis: Write a sentence of your choice. Provide dotted line.   1
Copy this shape as best you can alongside it[4].   1

1   Precede with 'I will mention 3 objects to you. Please repeat them to
    me once I have finished all 3.' Allow 1 s between objects.
    At end say 'I will ask you to remember these later' which is tested
    in Recall in next but one section – should be done after 1 min.
2   'Serial 7s' can also be used which obviously tests calculation too so
    remember to take into account premorbid numeracy skills.
3   Write out in large, clear capital letters 'CLOSE YOUR EYES'.
4   Only correct if makes 4-sided shape formed by
    2 intersecting pentagons.

- Allow 1 min for tasks, except 30 s for 3-stage command and
  writing of sentence.
- Score, 25/30 abnormal (i.e. dementia and/or delirium). 25–27 is
  borderline. *NB: frontal lobe tests not covered; useful to add.*

USEFUL FORMULAE

Serum osmolality $= 1.86\,(K^+ + Na^+) +$ urea + glucose
NB: all units are in *mmol/l* and this calculation is an *estimate* (actual
osmolality usually differs by ± 13 mosm/kg).

Anion gap $= (Na^+ + K^+) - (Cl^- + HCO_3^-)$
Normal range 8–16 mEq/l
$>16 =$ loss of HCO_3^- w/o concurrent increase in Cl^-.

Creatinine clearance $=$ [Urine creatinine] $\times$ urine flow rate/[Plasma
creatinine]

Body mass index $=$ Weight (kg)/height (m)^2
'Normal' (target) $= 18.5–25$

Weight conversions:

- 1 kg = 1000 g; 1 g = 1000 mg; 1 mg = 1000 micrograms;
  1 microgram = 1000 nanograms
- 1 stone = 6.35 kg; 1 kg = 2.2 lb.

COMMON LABORATORY REFERENCE VALUES

NB: normal ranges often vary between laboratories. The ranges given here are deliberately narrow to minimise missing abnormal results, but this means that your result may be normal for your laboratory's range, which should always be checked if possible.

Biochemistry

Na^+	135–145 mmol/l
K^+	3.5–5.0 mmol/l
Urea	2.5–6.5 mmol/l
Creatinine	70–110 µmol/l
Ca^{2+}	2.15–2.65 mmol/l
PO_4	0.8–1.4 mmol/l
Albumin	35–50 g/l
Protein	60–80 g/l
Mg^{2+}	0.75–1.0 mmol/l
Cl^-	95–105 mmol/l
Glucose (fasting)	3.5–5.5 mmol/l
LDH	70–250 iu/l
CK	25–195* u/l (↑in blacks)
Trop I	<0.4 ng/ml (= µg/l)
Trop T	<0.1 ng/ml (= µg/l)
D-dimers	<0.5** mg/l
Bilirubin	3–17 µmol/l
ALP	30–130 iu/l
AST	3–31 iu/l

*Sex differences exist: females occupy the lower end of the range.

**D-dimer normal range can vary with different test protocols: check with your lab.

Biochemistry (*Continued*)

ALT	3–35 iu/l
GGT	7–50* iu/l
Amylase	0–180 u/dl
Cholesterol	3.9–5.2 mmol/l
Triglycerides	0.5–1.9 mmol/l
LDL	<2.0 mmol/l
HDL	0.9–1.9 mmol/l
Urate	0.2–0.45 mmol/l
CRP	0–10 mg/l

Haematology

Hb male	13.5–17.5 g/dl
Hb female	11.5–15.5 g/dl
Pt	150–400 $\times 10^9$/l
WCC	4–11 $\times 10^9$/l
NØ	2.0–7.5 $\times 10^9$/l (40–75%)
LØ	1.3–3.5 $\times 10^9$/l (20–45%)
EØ	0.04–0.44 $\times 10^9$/l (1–6%)
PCV (5 Hct)	0.37–0.54* l/l
MCV	76–96 fl
ESR	<age in years (*+10 in women*)/2
HbA$_{1C}$	2.3–6.5%

*Sex differences exist: females occupy the lower end of the range.

Clotting

APTT	35–45 s
APTT ratio	0.8–1.2
INR	0.8–1.2

Haematinics

Iron	11–30 μmol/l
Transferrin	2–4 g/l
TIBC	45–72 μmol/l
Serum folate	1.8–11 μg/l
B_{12}	200–760 pg/ml (5 ng/l)

Arterial blood gases

PaO_2	> 10.6 kPa
$PaCO_2$	4.7–6.0 kPa
pH	7.35–7.45
HCO_3^-	24–30 mmol/l
Lactate	0.5–2.2 mmol/l
Base xs	± 2 mmol/l

Thyroid function

Thyroxine (total T_4)	70–140 nmol/l
Thyroxine (free T_4)	9–22 pmol/l
TSH	0.5–5 mU/l

INDEX

Adult tachycardia (with pulse) algorithm

European Resuscitation Council Guidelines 2010

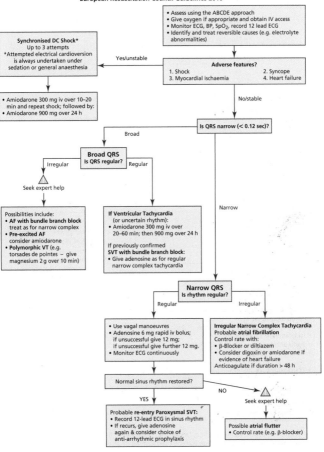

- Assess using the ABCDE approach
- Give oxygen if appropriate and obtain IV access
- Monitor ECG, BP, SpO₂, record 12 lead ECG
- Identify and treat reversible causes (e.g. electrolyte abnormalities)

Adverse features?
1. Shock
2. Syncope
3. Myocardial ischaemia
4. Heart failure

Yes/unstable

Synchronised DC Shock*
Up to 3 attempts
*Attempted electrical cardioversion is always undertaken under sedation or general anaesthesia

- Amiodarone 300 mg iv over 10–20 min and repeat shock; followed by:
- Amiodarone 900 mg over 24 h

No/stable

Is QRS narrow (< 0.12 sec)?

Broad

Broad QRS
Is QRS regular?

Irregular

Seek expert help

Possibilities include:
- **AF with bundle branch block** treat as for narrow complex
- **Pre-excited AF** consider amiodarone
- **Polymorphic VT** (e.g. torsades de pointes – give magnesium 2 g over 10 min)

Regular

If **Ventricular Tachycardia**
(or uncertain rhythm):
- Amiodarone 300 mg iv over 20–60 min; then 900 mg over 24 h

If previously confirmed
SVT with bundle branch block:
- Give adenosine as for regular narrow complex tachycardia

Narrow

Narrow QRS
Is rhythm regular?

Regular

- Use vagal manoeuvres
- Adenosine 6 mg rapid iv bolus; if unsuccessful give 12 mg; if unsuccessful give further 12 mg.
- Monitor ECG continuously

Normal sinus rhythm restored?

YES

Probable re-entry Paroxysmal SVT:
- Record 12-lead ECG in sinus rhythm
- If recurs, give adenosine again & consider choice of anti-arrhythmic prophylaxis

Irregular

Irregular Narrow Complex Tachycardia
Probable **atrial fibrillation**
Control rate with:
- β-Blocker or diltiazem
- Consider digoxin or amiodarone if evidence of heart failure
Anticoagulate if duration > 48 h

NO

Seek expert help

Possible atrial flutter
- Control rate (e.g. β-blocker)

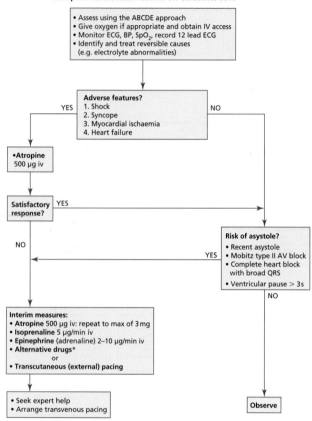

Adult bradycardia algorithm

European Resuscitation Council UK Guidelines 2010

- Assess using the ABCDE approach
- Give oxygen if appropriate and obtain IV access
- Monitor ECG, BP, SpO₂, record 12 lead ECG
- Identify and treat reversible causes
  (e.g. electrolyte abnormalities)

Adverse features?
1. Shock
2. Syncope
3. Myocardial ischaemia
4. Heart failure

YES / NO

- Atropine
  500 µg iv

Satisfactory response? — YES

NO

Risk of asystole?
- Recent asystole
- Mobitz type II AV block
- Complete heart block
  with broad QRS
- Ventricular pause > 3s

YES / NO

Interim measures:
- Atropine 500 µg iv: repeat to max of 3 mg
- Isoprenaline 5 µg/min iv
- Epinephrine (adrenaline) 2–10 µg/min iv
- Alternative drugs*
  or
- Transcutaneous (external) pacing

- Seek expert help
- Arrange transvenous pacing

Observe

*Alternatives include: Aminophylline, Dopamine, Glucagon (if β-blocker or Ca⁺⁺ channel blocker overdose) or Glycopyrrolate (can be used instead of atropine)